ROUTLEDGE LIBRARY EDITIONS:
EPISTEMOLOGY

Volume 14

THE SENSORY BASIS AND STRUCTURE OF KNOWLEDGE

THE SENSORY BASIS AND STRUCTURE OF KNOWLEDGE

HENRY J. WATT

Routledge
Taylor & Francis Group
LONDON AND NEW YORK

First published in 1925

This edition first published in 2015
by Routledge
2 Park Square, Milton Park, Abingdon, Oxon OX14 4RN

and by Routledge
605 Third Avenue, New York, NY 10017

Routledge is an imprint of the Taylor & Francis Group, an informa business

British Library Cataloguing in Publication Data
A catalogue record for this book is available from the British Library

ISBN: 978-1-138-80196-7 (Set)
ISBN: 978-1-315-69475-7 (Set) (ebk)
ISBN: 978-1-138-90432-3 (Volume 14) (hbk)
ISBN: 978-1-315-69461-0 (Volume 14) (ebk)

DOI: 10.4324/9781315694610

Publisher's Note
The publisher has gone to great lengths to ensure the quality of this reprint but points out that some imperfections in the original copies may be apparent.

Disclaimer
The publisher has made every effort to trace copyright holders and would welcome correspondence from those they have been unable to trace.

THE SENSORY BASIS AND STRUCTURE OF KNOWLEDGE

BY

HENRY J. WATT, D.PHIL.

METHUEN & CO. LTD.
36 ESSEX STREET W.C.
LONDON

First Published in 1925

PRINTED IN GREAT BRITAIN

PREFACE

THIS book is meant to serve as a short introduction to the systematic psychology of cognition, beginning with the study of its foundations in the simplest sensations, and following the process of complication onwards as far as the concept. This point seems to me to form a convenient and natural break. The exposition of all that other part of cognition that involves the concept is to a very large extent practically independent of the work of sensation, with which this book is concerned. Very little further light would be thrown upon the scheme of integration I have proposed by a sketch of its extension into the conceptual reaches of cognition. This practical cleavage between sensation and conception is already widely recognised. It accounts for the relative independence of logic, which begins and ends with the concept, so that it may be called the general science of the concept. It equally accounts for the power of psychoanalysis to flourish in spite of the fantastic theories of mind promulgated by its exponents. For it also is largely a kind of logic (of conceptual desire), which can likewise afford to ignore, or to be ignorant of, the real minutiæ of the mind's composition and their connexions, in short of psychology.

But, nevertheless, it has always been perfectly clear to those who pursue the problems of the actual data of mind and its elaboration that sensation and concept can never finally be taken as separate sources of mind. Sense must run smoothly and continuously into intellect. And there must be a regular process of integration leading from the elements and details of sensation, which the experimentation of the last fifty years has explored so minutely and fully, to the processes of thought whose elucidation seems so perplexingly difficult and as baffling to modern experimental investigation as to all other analyses of it of any time. Surely we must expect to find that only in so far as some basal scheme of exposition is accurately fitted on to the well-defined facts of sensation, so that we can carry it steadily forward through their complications, will the higher reaches of mind come under the scientist's control. We have all seen how true this is in chemistry. And I have always thought that there is a great similarity between the general outlook of the work, and the progress of chemistry and the psychology of cognition.

The book also presents a general exposition of the pure psychology of sensory experience that I have developed from time to time during the last fifteen years. A series of papers were published in the *British Journal of Psychology:* (1) "Some Problems of Sensory Integration," 1910, Vol. **3,** 323–347; (2) "The Elements of Experience and their Integration, or Modalism," 1911, **4,** 127–204; (3) "The Psychology of Visual Motion," 1913, **6,** 26–43; (4) "The Main Principles of Sensory Integration," 1913, **6,** 239–260; (5) "Psychological Analysis and Theory of Hearing," 1914, **7,** 1–43; (6) "Stereoscopy as a Purely Visual, Bisystemic, Integrative Process," 1916, **8,** 131–169; (7) "A Theory of Binaural Hearing," 1920, **11,** 163–171; and also "The Importance of the Sensory Attribute of Order, in Mind," 1920, **29,** 257–276. My book on the *Psychology of Sound* (Cambridge, 1917), is a detailed study of this analysis and theory of hearing, while the *Foundations of Music* (Cambridge, 1920), shows its very satisfactory agreement with the results of musical analysis and theory as commonly taught in textbooks of harmony and the like. Minor sketches of the plan of sensory integration have also been given in *Psychology* (T. Nelson and Sons, 1913), and *sub verbo* "Psychology" in *Hastings' Encyclopædia of Religion and Ethics*.

This book is, therefore, rather a thesis than a textbook. It promulgates a comparative method of analysis of sensory experience and a scheme of its progressive complication from the elements of sensation up to the primitive form of the concept. And it can claim not merely to be a distinctive method and theory, but to have already demonstrated its power to reduce the apparent confusion of sensory experience and to accelerate the successful analysis and systematic arrangement of many otherwise baffling facts.

I am emboldened now to publish a general statement of it because constant reflexion fails to shake my trust in the validity of its outlook and method. Expositions of the psychology of cognition are already numerous. But while they traverse the same ground, on the whole, their arrangements are very different: and they seem to lack entirely any general principle of procedure by which some agreement between them might be attained. An ever varying amount of physiology is mingled with the exposition, so that it may be quite hard for the beginner to see that he is really studying psychology rather than physiology, and certainly difficult for him to know where the physiology ends and psychology begins. Such interfused treatment of different spheres of descriptive facts, however dependent they may ultimately be on one another, cannot be favourable to complete and systematic statement of the psychological side. For long the various facts of sensory psychology have been set out so casually that the senses seemed to be utterly different and unconnected functions, severally subject to the most surprising complications, and to engender, or be subdued by, thought as by some miracle. The inevitable force of this impression made the effort to attain some sort of continuity of statement a constant despair. And so the only course seemed to be to postpone any such statement until by careful scrutiny of fact and cautious generalisation some approximate constancy of arrangement could be devised. The papers and books I have referred to mark the course of this work. In the meantime great progress in experimental study of sensation has been made which has filled up many gaps and transitions, and has made many analogies far more convincing than they could have been in themselves. But on the whole they have all tended to support the general sketch of the plan of rearrangement with which I began (*Br. J. Psych.*, Vol. 4, 1911).

Although a scheme of mental integration must seem speculative to most minds, I believe that the notion of it I have propounded contains nothing that is not functional or descriptive fact, even in so far as it does not attempt to reduce the negative element in the notion to any positive determination. That "something new" occurs under certain conditions seems at present an inference that may be escaped only at the risk of fantastic empiricism, or *ad hoc* speculation. If we can avoid it later on, then integration may become the name for the process then discovered. It should be a safe proceeding to sketch a hypothesis of analysis or integration on the basis of the simpler senses, and to test it in the more complex ones, estimating its probability by enumeration in the end and awaiting the light of further experimentation, as I have striven to do. Anyone who does not like the term integration, may ignore it, if he will, keeping only the systematic arrangement of the topics as a common framework of complication. There will be no real harm done even if he calls each integration a new sensation. For the great need in psychology is some agreed frame of exposition round which research may progressively accrete its results. The theory of mind will gradually make the dry bones of the frame live.

In recent years other parts of psychology have made great progress. But we may be sure that no extensions or changes of interest will ever suffice to eclipse the value and importance of the psychology of cognition. It will survive all our devotion to the interests of the individual, and all our concern for the practical issues of mind in conduct. No pragmatism of any kind will rob it of its life and existence. On the contrary, these other interests will sooner or later return to it for help in solving the central mystery of their own spheres. And, of course, there are disciplines of the most ideal practicality that are deeply interested in the pure science of cognition—physiology, logic, epistemology, æsthetics, to mention only a few. The well-spring of any "emergent" philosophy must surely be this field of our study in which alone we can observe and pursue the progressive steps of a series of "emergents" and from which alone we can venture to infer anything whatever about the possible "emergents" that constitute the rest of the world. My views on these questions I have attempted to indicate at various points, and especially in the last chapter.

I have tried to avoid the sentimental belittlement of rival theories and even of other branches of psychology that is so fashionable at present amongst the most diverse psychological schools. For however we may differ in the fields we choose to study and in the schemes of construction we prefer, we are all out for one and the same end—to ascertain the facts and to devise and secure the surest inferences. And all fields of psychology must progress together for the best welfare of each. There can be no differences which mere sentiment or moral superiority alone could guarantee. A value in science can never be moral or æsthetic or even practical: it can only be veridical. And if so, it is either present or absent. If it is present it will declare itself by its own power; no amount of terminological abuse of other theories will give it force. There is only one anathema that can be set upon a professed psychology: namely, that it is evidently non-psychological, whether it be physiological, logical, educational, industrial, physical or what not. It must be concerned with mind, by itself or in some setting. And then the only questions are: are the facts true, the inferences cogent, and the hypotheses safe?

H. J. W.

CONTENTS

THE SENSORY BASIS AND STRUCTURE OF KNOWLEDGE

CHAPTER I

INTRODUCTORY

THE primary task of psychology is to study the soul or the mind or experience or whatever you like to call it, so long as you mean what has from time immemorial been called mental or spiritual, sensation or thought, emotion or memory, action or passion, or anything similar to them or continuous with them. It is not the task of psychology at all to study matter and its functions, whether that matter is animate or inanimate, so long as it is not at the same time held to be actually or virtually mental. And this latter task belongs to it only as the study of neighbouring fields or common territory belongs to any science. In so far as we eliminate mind or "consciousness" from our interests altogether, the study of pure behaviour belongs properly to the field of physiology, which is concerned primarily with the functions of the animate organism, whether in parts by abstraction, or as a whole integrated unity. And in actual exposition the bias of the study of behaviour falls heavily towards the physiological pole. The centre of gravity of any study called psychology must lie in the mind.

In so far as any science keeps systematically and closely to its own field of interests, it is a "pure" science. When it passes into fields in which its special interests mingle with those of neighbouring sciences, it becomes an "applied" science. Thus, since the primary interest of psychology is mind, the systematic study and formulation of the structure and functions of mind itself constitutes pure psychology. The study of mind-controlled behaviour is still psychology to be sure; but it is, strictly, applied psychology. It is the outcome of the interest that pure psychology naturally extends to any events in which mind plays a decisive part. There is indeed a field of interest to which the name Behaviour may usefully be applied. And there may well form itself around this field a group of special students of Behaviour. But the group can never become exclusive and distinct from those of physiologists and of psychologists. For every applied science, every science of complex events, must attach itself more or less closely and pre-eminently to one pure science. The study of behaviour will devolve upon psychologists or upon those whose chief training has been psychological, in proportion to the prominence or importance of mental functions in behaviour. If the bodily functions or causes are more in question, the bias of the study will be towards pure physiology.

The direction of interest from behaviour towards physiology appears to be opposed to that towards psychology, because Mind and Matter are so very different realms. No doubt all parts and phases of the universe are equally objective in a philosophical sense. And no doubt, too, they are all continuous with one another and interdependent. But no logical device has yet succeeded in removing the division between the world of mind or phenomena and the world of matter or reality. The more we study the two in relation to one another the more definite are the traces we find of a parallelism of contact between them. At the same time the greater is the apparent difference between the things thus set into parallel. The great difference, too, between the forms of combination and interaction of the units of matter and those of experiences implies very different kinds of interest in those who devote themselves to their study.

This is broadly the difference between the engineer and the artist, between the mechanist and the æsthetist. The study of nature reduces itself ultimately and typically to dynamics or to mathematical physics. The study of mind revolves essentially on the study of mental synthesis and the new essence that this creates, which in the work of the artist is the beauty of a combination. The terms truth and goodness, to which some venture to add religion,[1] refer to the other great fields of spiritual synthesis and their resulting "light." These fields no doubt each include a great array of different steps of synthesis, equally unique and creative. But everyone who is acquainted with them knows that truth, beauty, and goodness are typically spiritual lights that have no "objective" counterpart in nature. We know absolutely nothing of any "light" of synthesis in nature, whereas in the world of mind we know practically nothing but this light. The dynamics of the synthesis itself, even the spiritual dynamics of it, remains almost wholly clouded in mystery.

The best philosophy of our day is undoubtedly that which is incorporated in the great and progressive schemes of the various sciences, physical, natural, and mental. There can be no philosophy of nature, such as our sciences have developed, without a corresponding philosophy of mind, even though the former seems to define the latter only by exclusion and neglect. Still it is that which the sciences of nature have found abiding reason to exclude from their system. And though negative, that is an excellent reason why we should anticipate systematic cohesion in the field so excluded. Psychology will do well, we may be sure, to attach itself generally to this great scheme of things and to strive to extend it or to modify it by supplementing it and thereby reacting upon it.

Many other schemes of being have been propounded by philosophers; but they remain essentially tentative and speculative. They are mere sketches or programs, inferior by the very fact that they have not succeeded in penetrating the actual work of science and remoulding it in detail to their new principles. To those who are trying to extend knowledge as well as to reform it as opportunity and insight allow, they may seem little more than visionary. It is a mistake to suppose that the work of philosophy differs from science in method and matter. Philosophy is nothing but the finally satisfactory scheme of all science. And the great scheme of the sciences is essentially the work of

[1] B. Bosanquet, *Some Suggestions in Ethics*, p. 68. London, 1919.

the philosophy of all the ages, to which the critical and constructive efforts of modern philosophers are as necessary as the research which so constantly extends it. There can therefore be no question as to the assumptions and presuppositions from which psychology will set out to review and arrange its subject-matter. In its own fields, of course, psychology is absolutely free of every prejudice. In relation to the fields that surround it, it must enter into sympathetic contact with the schemes that they adopt.

It is more necessary now than ever that emphasis should be laid upon the pure and systematic ideal of psychology. Physiological and psychological interests have not always been so clearly defined and distinguished as they should have been, so that considerable obscurity and confusion of purposes were inevitable.[1] The pursuit of psychological problems has often failed because physiological results seemed more promising and "objective." The physiological issues of psychological study seemed at first to be an extension of psychology itself and a welcome relief from the difficulties of a pure and systematic psychology. Hence the apparent substantiality and the considerable popularity of "Physiological Psychology." The gradual accompanying conquest of the field by experimental methods was undoubtedly an enormous and permanent benefit to psychology. But we must now review the situation and recognise that physiological references add nothing whatever to the field of psychological knowledge, no matter how correct and valuable they may be in themselves. They are essentially foreign, even though neighbouring territory. The perennial problem of the study of mind in terms of itself remains unobscured through all advances of knowledge. And it can be finally and completely successful only in so far as the realm of mind remains autonomous territory, and as such enters into alliance with the realms around it.

In recent years so great advances have been made in the various fields of applied psychology that the distracting effect of contact with physiology has been increased a

[1] Cf. the article "Psychology," in *Hastings' Encyclop. of Religion and Ethics*, Vol. X, 424 f.

hundredfold. A systematist in psychology now seems to be somewhat of a rarity. Expositions of "Objective Psychology," of systems of "Behaviour," and other such formulations grow more and more numerous. An attempt has even been made to declare the non-existence of mind, consciousness, and all such "myths." Psychology, of course, can only ultimately gain by the renewal of zeal that comes from every advance it makes as an applied science. And it is possible that the area of its applications will finally bulk very large in the total sphere of influence of the science. But no pure science can be annulled by any such changes in its surroundings. Sciences are not like fashions that die for lack of love. They never die. And they are content to wait till any novelty becomes familiar, confident that the true perspective will be restored before long. If there is one thing in the world that is insuppressible it is mind. The meteoric brilliance of the physical sciences failed to crush it, though it made mind seem isolated and impotent. Even the future culmination of cerebral physiology will not render it lifeless. There is matter in the world, no doubt, to set against all the mind it contains. But there is mind as well. A picture or a statue is in itself completely material. But both of them were made for their beauty. And surely no one fancies that music can ever be bought or broken, though the means to it may be so handled.

It is long since Sherrington and others first braced up the systematic and direct study of the nervous system into pure and constructive science. Physiology is now thoroughly permeated by the direct and exclusive ideal of exposition in terms of organism and function. The nervous system is set forth as if no mind were connected with it all. The time is due when psychology, too, should set its house in order and sweep it clear of physiological litter. The mind must be laid out in terms of its own elements and their combinations and integrations. Physiological information and psychophysical inferences may be added to any desired extent. But the demarcation between them and what is psychological should be perfectly clear, so that any poverty of fact or finish in the latter may be evident.

In order to make this demarcation perfectly clear, the following rather elementary distinctions may be permitted. A psychological proposition is one that has for its subject some experience or mental process, and for its predicate some quality or property thereof or some relation to another experience or some term of quantity, and so on. " Warmth and cold are different kinds of sensation," " the octave is a better fusion than the fifth," " there are two feelings, pleasure and displeasure," are examples. It is the primary aim of psychology to increase the number of exact and true psychological propositions and to make them as systematic and complete as possible.

Physiology is concerned with the parts of the body and their functions. And on this basis its work is analogous to that of psychology. " The eye is the receptor of light," and " there is one set of spots on the skin receptive to temperatures of low degree and another receptive to those of relatively high degree " are purely physiological propositions.

But as the mind and the body are dependent upon one another, these two sciences have to be brought into correlation with one another in a science that may generally be called psychophysics. Examples of psychophysical propositions are : " the eye is the sense-organ of vision," " no special organs for pleasure and displeasure have yet been discovered," " there is one set of receptors in the skin for cold and one for warmth." It is possible, of course, to claim that the " sense-organ of vision " means the anatomical eye, and that cold and warmth are physical terms. But physiology and Behaviour know of nothing but light, and physics deals only with temperatures, not with cold and warmth. The sentence referring to cold and warmth conveys the idea that different material bodies are responsible for sensations or " feelings " that as such are different apart from any knowledge of body whatever. And vision is the world we have " before us " when the eye is excited to function by light.

This use of the term psychophysics differs slightly from current usage. But the limitation of the word to the relation between differences of sensation and changes in the physical stimuli that evoke them is rather too special and historical to be necessary. The extension of meaning we imply seems not only to be useful, but to correspond to the modern use of the term "physical," to include the fundamental processes of animate as well as of inanimate nature. Psychophysics remains the same sort of science whether experiences are related to the central nervous system and its parts along with the peripheral receptors, or to the quantitative changes of stimuli necessary to provoke their graded differences. The former relation is commonly called psychophysiology, or physiological psychology; but it really includes the latter relation. The older term psychophysics has also the great merit of brevity.

Therefore these three terms—physiology, psychology, and psychophysics—cover the whole ground of pure and applied psychology and the surrounding area of organism. Any further systematic terms can only lead to confused ideas regarding what is essentially simple. It seems incredible that students of psychology should spend so much time talking and writing about the definition of their science and should feel impelled to wonder whether in the future Behaviourism or Introspectionism will get the upper hand or occupy the field. We might as well discuss whether finally mechanical inventions or the old-fashioned process of artistic creation will dominate music. Introspection is merely a name for the observation of the mental. The total suppression of the word could only lead to greater clarity in the principles of psychology. There can be no competition between the observation of the mental and the study of the stimuli, responses and intervening changes in the organism. We separate the studies of mind and body not only because we can, but because we must. But we can therefore combine them afterwards in any relative mixture we may find serviceable. This may be called by any characteristic name, but it is in any case psychophysics in its systematic nature.

Thus Industrial Psychology is for the most part a physiological, or even physical, investigation. It seeks to establish the conditions of greatest efficiency—greatest labour in average unit-time of work—of the human machine. It does not necessarily attend to the state of mind of the worker, whether active or resting. The same principles of investigation would suit any other machine whose efficiency was restrained (by overheating, vibration or other conditions) to a moderate maximum. But Industrial Psychology in its general scope does include consideration of the feelings, the interests, the satisfaction of the worker; it has some account with pure psychology. It is essentially a Psychological Physiology, though that term is too abstract to serve as a useful designation for it. Nevertheless, the term is systematically correct, and that is our particular interest at the moment. Industrial Psychology is a branch of psychophysics.

Psychoanalysis, on the contrary, is a part of pure psychology. It assumes and believes, at least so far as the complex mind of the thinking individual is concerned, that mind is a closed system of interacting processes, forming normally an orderly realm of associative ideas or complexes. By the action of primary sources of accretion in unusual strength and by the resulting conflicts a disorderly state of mind can ensue. Various devices enable us to restore this mind to order again, and thereby the disorder that had been apparent in conduct is automatically removed. It is assumed herewith that the relations between mind and body are in themselves stable and unambiguous. The interest of psychoanalysis in the physical side of conduct is purely negative or negligible. It consists in the determination by the physician himself, or by another person who is a physician, that the subject shows no physical symptoms.

The older pathology of mind held the still prevalent view that all disorders of mind were merely the reflexion through the psychophysical nexus of primary disturbances of the organism. It was tacitly assumed that mind in itself is always inert and passively perfect. It is at every moment set by conditions that are "external" to it or physical, and it always of itself completes without defect or disorder every process of change or complication to which it is thus set. It does not initiate any process of change, whether of relations or of forces, or any synthesis or dissociation entirely by itself. It is, of course, extremely difficult to refute this theory. And it would be wrong to suppose that psychoanalysis has done so in any particular case. This discipline is satisfied in showing how often and how swiftly apparently grievous disorders of conduct, that seem merely to be of physical origin, are removed by treatment of the patient's mind. It infers that the disorder of conduct in such cases had its origin in mental disorder. Against this, we find the serious claim that similar disorders of the mind can be removed by thoroughly ridding the body of all focal infections, when the mind as automatically resumes its orderly course.[1] Whichever of these theories may ultimately prevail, the purely psychological standpoint adopted by psychoanalysis will surely persist and retain its own relative value as an easy, direct, and often sufficient, method.

Of their own nature and according to the opinion of the vast majority of psychologists experiences fall into three groups. (1) The sensory-cognitive system includes all sensations and their complexities, perception, conception, imagination, memory, thought, reasoning, and the like. (2) The emotive system includes all non-sensory feelings, especially pleasure and displeasure, all the emotions such as fear, anger, love, and all the sentiments, such as reverence, dignity and gratitude, etc. (3) The conative system includes the work of the appetites, such as hunger and sex, the "instinctive" expression of emotion, the expression of voluntary decisions, and so on.

It is, of course, impossible to study these three systems in complete isolation from one another. They interweave continually with one another in every moment of life. But to a large extent they can be treated separately. The sensory-cognitive system, for example, stands for many purposes, apart from the emotive system and even from the conative too. We try to hear, see, perceive, and think correctly and exactly without the interference of our emotions and our prejudiced wills, even although there may be no wholly unmotivated cognition. Scientific observation must be exact in its dependence upon the agreed circumstances, which are nearly always physical, and it must be impartial. It must consist of cognitive

[1] Cotton, H. A., *The Defective, Delinquent and Insane.* London, 1921.

processes that under these circumstances are inevitable and so universal. If any system of mind may legitimately be abstracted from the rest, it is the sensory-cognitive one.

But the emotive system would be all " in the air " if it were isolated from the sensory-cognitive system. Our feelings and sentiments would be all about nothing whatever. The study of this system should, therefore, in principle follow, and be set into relation to, a temporarily satisfactory study of the sensory-cognitive one. Similarly our actions would be senseless if we acted for no reason or purpose and without enthusiasm of any kind. So the study of action follows naturally upon that of the two others.

In every study we may proceed in either of two ways: we may pass either from the simple to the complex, or from the complex to the simple. The former method is generally followed by the natural sciences, such as chemistry or biology. In them it has the advantage of displaying not only the logical complication of the subject, but also in many respects the development of things studied—the individual organism, the animal kingdom, the world of organic substances. But it would be wrong to suggest that there is any strict parallel between the course of real development and of systematic exposition. The other method has the merit of showing the start and progress of knowledge itself. Our first acquaintance is with the complicated organisms and substances of our world. By patient enquiry and experiment we learn to reduce them to complexes of simpler parts whose properties seem to be more general and uniform than those of the earlier known objects.

Both these methods have been followed in psychology, " Simple to complex " gives the exposition the form of a synthesis of elements, especially in the sensory-cognitive system. There it has the same advantages as in the natural sciences. It presupposes more or less successful analysis and gives proper emphasis to the problems of synthesis that alone show the completeness of knowledge. Logically this implies frequent use of the method of deduction in which the array of one set of facts enables the reader to anticipate other sets of facts that have been supplied by systematic experimentation and that thus appear as complications of the first set. And the method corresponds in general to the probable course of the complication of cognition in the animal kingdom.

" Complex to simple " is more tender to the beginner in psychology, leading him from the familiar terms of his daily experience gently towards the farther reaches of the scientist's analysis. And there are some who hold that this method is true to the probable course of development of cognition—from a large " undifferentiated continuum " of feeling to the details of distinction that we adults carry out so easily in everyday life. But this view can hardly escape the charge of vagueness.

We shall adopt the method of synthesis, hoping that our success with it may help to justify it. Apart from the problem of development—and the natural sciences indicate that that proceeds very often at least from the simple to the complex, we can lose nothing by working in this direction. It is easier to analyse boldly and widely, as experiment typically does, and then to study carefully whether our results can be put together so as to display the whole nature and essence of the sensory experience we meet with daily, than it is to refrain from the least analysis until we are sure that we have omitted no step that led us to the grade of analysis we have at any moment reached. There are minds, to be sure, that so love the currents and pulses of daily life that they are repelled by the strange elements and forces that science claims to reveal in its structure. But these are not the minds for whom science is constructed.

CHAPTER II

THE ELEMENTS OF SENSATION

THE OUTER SENSES

FOR the purpose of systematic study it is convenient and useful to divide the senses into three groups.

The first includes the senses spread generally over the surface of the body and in certain other parts. These may be called the outer senses, and they are primarily the senses of pain, touch, cold, and warmth. Their psychological character is relatively clear and simple. They set before us a pattern that we may attempt to verify and to apply to the elucidation of the other senses. The need for a class of special cutaneous senses not generally spread over the skin is doubtful.

The senses of the second group are found either in the middle substance of the body (especially in or near the muscles and the joints) or on the inner surface of the body (the alimentary canal and its adjuncts); so they may be called the inner senses. They include mainly the muscular, articular, and the "organic" sensations. Their psychological character and status, even their mere existence, is still in question. They may, therefore, be deemed to be obscure, but they need not be considered to be specially complicated. Their obscurity is doubtless the result of their inaccessibility and their poor physiological variation.

The third includes the higher senses of hearing, vision, smell, and taste. These are surely the most difficult and complicated of all. The sense of taste is comparatively simple, although it shares certain characteristics of the others. It may be treated as a link to carry us back to the first group. For a tongue-sense may be considered without extravagance as a (special) skin-sense.

This classification of the senses may claim to be both

methodical and fruitful. It seems better to begin with relatively simple and clear senses, to pass to those that are still simple though obscure, and to finish by applying the results of our study as a hypothesis for the elucidation of complicated and difficult senses. The contrary course, however, is far commoner probably because the senses of vision and hearing offer more details for exposition, and appeal more easily to the interests of the student. But this procedure distorts the scientific status of these senses and leads to neglect not only of the other senses, but of the systematic coherence of all the senses. Besides the method now followed—a comparative and systematic method—has actually led to the elucidation of the sense of hearing in a way that was never hitherto attempted,[1] and that may be said to have shown the complete conformity of this sense to the type common to the majority of the senses and patent enough in the cutaneous senses. A method that has been so fruitful should be applied all round, and may be expected to yield other results of importance if faithfully and diligently pursued. In any case, it is one that does more to ensure the systematic application to every sense of every problem that arises anywhere in any sense than does any other method, if there is any other notable one. It is, therefore, a method that provokes discovery. As such, it is applicable not only to the study of the elementary details of the senses, but to their complexities at any and every level of complication. And so it may be considered the method that most generally characterises the exposition of this book.

The study of sensory experience may, in fact, be said to offer two ideals for the guidance of investigation, namely (1) the thoroughgoing uniformity of all the senses in respect of their elements and at any level of complication in so far as they are complicated; and (2) the progressive and complete complication of their material in so far as the multiplication of this material in its most elementary form makes complication possible. We thus come in touch with the ideals that in the natural sciences have proved to be such potent and real forces, and that convert the patient

[1] Cf. *The Psychology of Sound*. Cambridge, 1917. *The Foundations of Music*. Cambridge, 1920.

groping of the collector and experimenter into an enlightened will that is conscious of the promise of what has been gained and can with each gain the more clearly estimate the completion of the task. When methods of this kind succeed, it means that the science that formerly was blind now begins to see.

It is a familiar fact that the whole surface of the body is dotted over with four sets of "spots," one of which is sensitive to warmth, one to cold, one to touch, and one to pain. These spots can readily be located by systematic exploration of an area with pointed stimuli of suitable kinds. They are scattered irregularly over the surface, being separated by varying gaps in which there is no sensitivity to the specific stimulus. The relative frequency of the spots of these four senses is very roughly thus: 0 to 3 per square centimetre for warmth, 6 to 23 for cold, 25 on the average for touch, and on a part of the back of the hand 100 to 200 for pain. On hairy parts, which form about 95 per cent of the whole surface of the body, there is a touch spot above the root of every hair. It is interesting to discuss possible reasons for the relative frequency indicated by these figures. They will naturally be of biological order.

From these sensory spots we get a natural element or particle of sensation. And it is important to consider what properties or attributes we may ascribe to this particle. Six important aspects or attributes have been distinguished.

(1) Quality.—The spots fall naturally into four classes or senses, according to the *kind* of sensation they evoke, whether warmth or cold or touch or pain. There is nothing again noticeably common to these four kinds; but we may say that they differ from one another in quality in so far as we make a group or class of these four kinds, for each of which we have familiar terms that are doubtless as old as speech itself. So these qualities are most obvious attributes.

(2) Intensity.—This is quite as patent to ordinary observation as quality and is familiar in each skin sense as the same sort of change, whether it be cold or pain or touch that is thus increasing. The intensity of a sensation can be greater or less, but it consists of no distinguishable

parts, more of which might be present in one sensation than in another of less intensity. The intensity of a sensation in other words, is a certain magnitude. And from a more or less definite minimal limit there seems to be a continuous gradation of intensity up to an indefinite maximal limit. A numerical value may be given to this intensity in terms of any natural or arbitrary numeration applied to this continuous series.

A natural unit, for instance, is found in the steps of just perceptible difference that may be marked out by careful statistical experiments on the discrimination of sensations. But it is clear that this natural step of difference can be recorded only in terms of the differences in the physical stimulus (applied to the organ) that is necessary on the average for the purpose of discrimination. We cannot say that one pain particle (from one spot) contains a less intense pain particle (from the same or any other spot) a certain number of times. Nor can we say it contains anything else a certain number of times, not even the minimal pain intensity or just noticeable difference. A severe pain contains nothing minimal in itself; it is simply severe, and as such obviously much greater than the minimal pain. Nor does it contain many differences in itself, for it is a pain, not a bunch or series of differences, implicit or explicit, between pains. But it is quite true to say that it is the $(n+1)$th pain, i.e. the pain that is just noticeably greater than the nth pain (which is the one just noticeably greater than the $(n-1)$th pain, and so on down to the first or minimal pain). This fact can be expressed quite as truly by saying that the pain is produced by a stimulus of such and such a physical pressure, the just noticeably less pain being produced by a certain smaller pressure, and so on. Neither method of recording steps for the series of pains tells us anything about the pains themselves.

Up to a certain point we can record the magnitude of a pain or a warmth in our memory and recognise its equal or greater again. Thus we carry with us an "absolute impression" or memory of its magnitude. But this absolute impression implies nothing more than is involved in the direct observation or comparison of any (intensive) magnitude. In every case we merely find for the magnitude more or less roughly a place in a series of continuous gradations of intensity.

Intensity, then, is a magnitude and cannot in any *direct* way be conceived as a multitude, i.e. as a unity containing in itself in some real sense many smaller units.[1] Myers,[2] it is true, has sought to establish on physiological grounds the theory that intensity is a kind of density of process. But, however much this interpretation may seem to suit the psychical nature of intensity, there are no facts of a psychological nature to support it. And so it remains on the psychical side nothing but a picture or parable of intensity, not yet a theory of it.

Increase of intensity of sensation is usually dependent upon quantitative increase of the stimulus. And, within the ordinary range of intensive differences, each step of just noticeable difference in the sensation involves increase of the stimulus by a constant ratio (Weber's law). Thus if a noise is made by dropping an ivory ball from a height upon an ebony plate, just noticeable differences in loudness will be produced on the average (or the like) by increase in the height of drop from 9 inches to 12, from 12 to 16, from 16 to 21·3 and so on, the ratio being four-thirds. Upon this basis Fechner (1801–1887) endeavoured to establish a law of the relation between psychical and physical magnitudes, namely, that as the stimulus to a sensation increases by some constant *ratio*, the corresponding sensation increases by some constant *amount*. This law assumes that the difference between the two sensations is itself a little bit of sensation, an amount that can be added, and has been added, to the smaller to make the greater sensation of the two. But there is no evidence of any kind that supports this assumption, as we have seen. The attempt has been made to test it by taking two very different sensations, A and C, and finding (1) the sensation B that will make the difference between A and B seem equal to that between B and C; and (2) determining the numbers of steps of just noticeable difference that separate A from B and B from C. If these two numbers are equal, the

[1] Cf. "Are the Intensity Differences of Sensations Quantitative," *Br. J. Psych.*, 1913, **6**, 175 ff.

[2] *Ibid.*, 1913, **6**, 137 ff.

steps of just noticeable difference will all be equal; for the two differences A—B and B—C are *presumably* really as well as apparently equal. Presumably! But the question is: are they really? We have not improved the argument at all by introducing the differences A—B and B—C. For they merely repeat the problem of the just noticeable difference. And we shall not make any progress in establishing such a psychophysical law until we have some purely psychological or direct evidence regarding quantity in sensation; or until we can state some quantitative (not merely enumerative) relation between sensations without using any physical facts in our argument at all. So long as our quantitative terms all remain on the physical side, we cannot transfer them to the psychical side. Mere enumeration of psychical differences or other units is not enough; for the primary question is whether these units are equal. Only then does the number of them become significant.

The physical basis of the Weber-Fechner law has been classified by reference to the analogous law (Nernst's) of the electrostatic potential difference, $\Phi_1 - \Phi_2$ of two concentrations of ions (C and C_2). According to Nernst's theory of galvanic chains, a sudden leap in the electrostatic potential takes place along the whole line, so that the single potentials mutually determine each other according to the expression $\Phi_1 - \Phi_2 = \text{const. log. } \frac{C_2}{C_1}$ which is in its form a parallel to Fechner's formula for Weber's law. We may suppose that two sensations, say two patches of colour, correspond to two cerebral areas between which there is an adjustment of the osmotic pressure on the part of the contained ions.[1] But it would be naïve to suppose that this illuminating explanation sheds any light at all upon the intensive relations of sensations as psychological entities. It does not give us any entry into the stuff of *sensations* at all.

No doubt there is some law in the relations between

[1] Cf. K. Koffka, "Perception: An Introduction to the Gestalt Theorie." *Psych. Bull.*, 1922, **19**, 531 ff. E. Becher, "W. Köhlers physikalische Theorie, etc." *Ztsch. f. Psych.*, 1921, **87**, 1 ff. W. Köhler, *Die physischen Gestalten in Ruhe und im stationären Zustande*, Brannschweig, 1920.

intensive differences of sensation and quantitative changes of the neural processes, whatever they are, that directly subserve them. Changes on the two sides will probably be "parallel" to one another. But we cannot state this law, if, as we see, we cannot measure psychical differences of intensity in themselves. If we could, we might be able to show by what rule physical energy or quantity is converted into, or is equivalent to, mental energy or magnitude. The notion of mental energy is now being freely manipulated in the popular literature of psychology: but it is quite a loose and vague notion, for no strict notion of mental or psychical energy or quantity has yet been established.

(3) Extent.—Many thinkers, following Descartes, have refused to attribute extent to anything mental. And no one seems ever to have held that thoughts have any mass or extension. Nevertheless, many sensations do seem to have extent, and especially the cutaneous sensations. Warmth and cold may be drop-like or massive like the warmth of a bath. Pain can be as fine as "pins and needles" or bulky like rheumatism or colic. A finger pressed upon the table gives a small extent of touch; the whole hand gives a large area. Some of the senses, such as smell and hearing, seem to offer no parallel to this. But we shall consider them more closely in their turn. The senses of the first group are undoubtedly extensive.

The "spot" of sensation seems in various respects to behave as if it were a minimal extent of sensation. For we cannot divide it into parts by any attitude of observation or by any physical change of stimulus. But it is possible that this particle may be reduced in extent, as when the intensity of the stimulus is decreased. And the sensory particle of some spots is smaller than of others. The miminal spot of pain is very small indeed, like the finest needle, the particle of touch is a good deal bigger, cold rather larger still, and warmth perhaps two or three times the size of that, on a rough estimate.

(4) Systemic position.—Two particles of cold may have the same quality, the same intensity, and the same extent, and yet be immediately distinguishable from one another, even if they appear and disappear simultaneously. This

difference corresponds, as everyone knows, to the physical "position" of each among the other cold spots of the skin. And so it may be called the attribute of position (or of "order" [1]) of the particle. Each particle of touch or pain we must suppose to be endowed with an inherent feature or attribute whereby it simply is a certain position. We do not give it its position by thinking about it or by attending to it. If it had no position, we could not give it one; and if its position is vague or indefinite we cannot alter it so as to make it more precise merely by thinking about it or noticing it. So the position of the particle is as much an inherent property or attribute of it as its intensity or its quality.

All the spots of warmth that can be evoked from the whole surface of the skin (and from other parts where they may occur) make up the sense of warmth. This system of spots corresponds to the system of organs in the skin that constitutes the sense of warmth physiologically. It is useful to have a term to specify this kind of (areal) system that is exemplified in nearly every sense. We shall therefore speak of the *systemic* attributes of extent and position.

It may seem strange that we can distinguish only one "position" in what is often quite a large spot of sensation, as warmth, for example, usually is. An attribute of position suggests the infinite distinction of positions that is so familiar in connexion with the points of mathematical systems. Of course we can think of the infinitely small or large in sensations as well as in any other kind of stuff. But we cannot by thought introduce marked or noticeable distinctions into things that do not present them. All we need for the present is some sort of picture of the spot of sensation that will enable us to see how these somewhat diverse attributes of position (ideally extentless) and of extent (ideally an infinity of positions) are reconcilable in a real thing. This picture we find in Bernstein's theory, according to which the spot is not a perfectly homogeneous area of sensation, but rather a circular mound of it, as it were. In the centre of the mound the intensity of the sensation is relatively greatest, and from there it falls

[1] Cf. *Br. J. Psych.*, 1911, **4**, 138 ff.

quickly and smoothly down to a vanishing quantity. To be observable it is well known that sensation must reach a certain minimal intensity. The extent of it that is really involved in any spot cannot therefore be fully covered by our observation, but only the more or less vaguely defined extent that is intense enough to be observable. And the position of the spot as a whole is not set by the only position it may conceivably contain, but by the position of its most intense part, its centre probably.

This interesting and important theory of the spot thus assumes the right to think of the spot of sensation in a mathematical way. A parallel assumption may be made for the subservient central excitation of neural process. But the psychological assumption is not here inferred from any physical facts alone. It is needed (systematically) first of all in order to explain the connexion between the extent and the position of the spot of sensation. And it implies a number of mathematical deductions of great value in the study of the complications of sensations. We shall discuss them in due course.

Instead of the attribute of position mention has often been made of an attribute of localisation. But localisation is obviously an operation that involves the reference or connexion of a sensation to something else—to the finger or hand or to our thought of it or to the sensations of some other sense by which we feel it. We refer a cold particle to a spot *on the skin*. But apart from this reference altogether the cold particle has inherent in it a feature that involves no process or reference, that simply is the position of the particle (amongst other particles) and that surely is the very means by which we become able to give it the reference we call localisation. It is a well-known fact that those who have lost a limb often feel pain " in the lost limb," as definitely located as it could be in any real limb. In the course of time this illusory localisation may grow more and more indefinite and vague. It may even be altered by " experience " to agree better with the state of the body. But such change of " correspondence," like the original learning of reference to the seen part, implies a constant basis of differentiation inherent in the sensation all the time, i.e. its systemic position.

(5) Duration.—Every sensation endures for some length of time, and so may be said to have the attribute of duration. Its duration, in other words, is a direct property of it, not a relation which we somehow establish as valid for it by the study of its connexion or dependence upon other things whose duration can be measured. The duration of a sensation is as much inherent in it as is its quality or intensity. This attribute forms a sort of parallel to the systemic attribute of extent. Both are kinds of continuous spread-out-ness, differing only in dimension, as it were. The dimension of duration is commonly called " temporal," and we have called the other " systemic " in order to distinguish it. Every duration, like every extent, is of a certain magnitude. But there is no naturally fixed particle of temporal extent, as there is of sensory extent in the sensory spot. The only other unit that may be suggested is the *just noticeable increment* of duration. But it has here again the disadvantage of not being a separable particle, but only an increment, i.e. a difference between two durations, judged to be so by cognition, not itself a detectable brief duration ; just as the difference between the literary value of two books or the prestige of two men is not itself a value or a reputation.

(6) Temporal position.—Like the minimal particle of sensory extent, every short duration shows an individual form of the sixth attribute of sensation, the temporal counterpart of systemic position. This attribute of temporal position suggests the same train of thought as we associated with systemic position. And an analogue to Bernstein's theory is already to hand in the facts that have been ascertained regarding the rise and fall of intensity in a sensation of brief duration. The sensation does not set in with maximal intensity. It begins minimal and quickly increases to a maximum, at which it dwells as long as may be, dying out rapidly thereafter. When identical sounds are made at regular intervals, this process of increase and decrease of intensity must give each of them as heard a more definite position than it otherwise might have. If the sounds were made more intense, each of them must appear to last longer, because it would then reach its maximum more quickly. And the time-interval

between loud sounds will appear shorter than between weaker sounds of the same physical rate of succession. Other deductions of importance can be made, notably those connected with the coalescence of sensations and their resulting intensity, a topic to which we shall return immediately.

Since both systemic and temporal extent are continuous and do not, as such, consist of noticeable and natural parts, it might be argued that positions in these two continuities are marked out only by the occurrence of qualities of sense with their intensities while the intervals (the distances and times) between them indirectly ensure that we shall attribute position to these qualities. Position would thus be the intellectual resultant of the apparent dissection of an essentially invariable and undissectable continuity by the appearance within it of quite different attributes, namely, quality and intensity. But this theory would not suffice to record the actual facts of sense. For both systemic distances and temporal intervals are magnitudes. And as such two distances or two times may be equal. If they were equal and nothing more than this, i.e. if they had not themselves a position in their respective dimensions which differentiated them from one another, there could be no proper field of form (" space "), or time, such as we actually find. We should not be able to observe that one distance lay here, the other there, or that one time came early, another later. This important property of these dimensions can only be secured by attributing a manifold of positions (with a real limit of distinction) both to the systemic and to the temporal continuity. The appearance of an intensive quality merely shows up or exposes a systemic position and a temporal position, if it is of small extent in these two dimensions. If it is of larger extent in either, that extent has a definite position in virtue of the manifold of unexposed positions which it must be held really to include in itself. Apart from particular exposure, however, this manifold remains merely potential in the continuity, while even so it definitely places the extent in its dimensions.[1]

[1] Cf. "The Importance of the Attribute of Order. *Mind*, **29**, 257 ff.

At the same time it is well to observe that the distinction of these six attributes has not been reached solely and simply by direct inspection of the elementary sensations themselves. Observation must, of course, confirm them. And it does so. But there is a long history behind their recognition, and many issues lie concealed within them that can only appear as we progress in our study of the complications of sensation. Every mode of integration of sensations, like every combination and reaction of chemical substances, raises problems regarding the nature of the elements, and persuades us to look for properties in them that might account for these higher powers. In sensation it is especially the problem of " space-perception " that has constantly renewed the discussion of the attributes of sensation. The argument has often been very long and involved [1] and leads in the end only a little more urgently towards the assumptions and observations involved in the attributes we have distinguished. So it seems better to remodel the exposition from the beginning to include both such observations as can be made directly upon the elements and such properties as we must assume in them in order to provide a basis for the higher structures of sense, and, it may be, of cognition as well. The exposition of psychology will for this reason constantly have to be reformed as our knowledge of the upper reaches of mind increases. The height and the depth of knowledge progress together. It will be evident as we proceed that space-perception is by no means the only problem in which the attributes of sensation play an important part. In fact, they ought never to be lost from sight, for they are the stuff of which cognition consists or upon which it is built. They are the warp and woof of its whole garment.

It was not until 1885 that the punctate distribution of the sensitivity of the skin was discovered by Blix and by Goldscheider. For all practical purposes our skin seems able to feel pain, touch, and temperature all over, although differences of sensitivity and of delicacy of discrimination are familiar to everyone. Thus the finger-tip is the special

[1] Cf. the treatment of it in Ladd and Woodworth's *Physiolog. Psychology*.

instrument of touch, the cheek and forearm of temperature, while the conjunctiva is extremely sensitive to pain. We know that a midge may bite without our feeling it, till the irritation of its poison spreads to the nearest pain-spot. But we never think that we are encased in a protective mail of the finest mesh for pain, " overlaid " by three others with progressively looser defences against their larger or diffuse stimuli. When we plunge the hand into water, the warmth seems to clothe it entirely ; it does not feel like a starry sky of points of warmth. And yet we must suppose that this mass of warmth consists of all the spots of warmth that we could find in the immersed part by the most careful exploration of it with a pointed metal rod. The many little particles of warmth together make up a large mass or volume of it. How shall we think of this fusion in detail ?

Here we can make good use of Bernstein's notion of intensive grading within the spot of sensation. When all the spots of an area are aroused, we shall have from each the sensation that we have from it when it alone is stimulated. But their outlying parts will now presumably overlap and so close up the continuity of the whole resultant. We shall no longer notice in the resultant area of sensation any of the points or relative maxima of the component spots, so long as we suppose the coalescence of the spots to be well balanced. But their fusion may very well produce some slight apparent increase or even decrease of intensity over the area. This will probably depend upon the intensity of stimulation of the spots or upon the relative number of spots in an area that are effectually stimulated. Generally the more extended the area continuously stimulated, the more intense is the sensation.

Thus for a certain degree of intensity of stimulation the overlap between neighbouring spots will just suffice to produce by summation an even level of intensity from the centre of the one spot to the other.[1] If the stimulation of both these spots is then made more intense, the overlap will probably be relatively more extensive than it was and so the total level of summation all over will be higher than

[1] Single spots do seem to be capable of different degrees of stimulation. K. Hansen, *Ztsch. Biol.*, 1921, **73**, 167 ff.

the central maximum of any contributing spot by itself. If the intensity is reduced, the overlap may be less extensive than before. And if there is any tendency for these simultaneous excitations physiologically to coalesce and to produce a common level (not in the peripheral sense-organs of course, but centrally), then the general level of intensity will be lower still. The limits of such processes of coalescence will, of course, vary from sense to sense. They must be much narrower, for example, in the sense of touch than in the senses of temperature or we should not be able to discriminate degrees of roughness as well as we do. But roughness is felt much better by the moving hand than by motionless pressure, as everyone knows.

We can now readily understand that when a large number of elementary particles of sensation of neighbouring position are evoked together, they will commonly fuse to form a continuous area of sensation. And in that area each element will help to determine along with its next neighbours the exact *conformation* of the areal sensation at the point at which it stands. If it is much more intense than its next neighbours, there will be an intensive prominence at that point of the area, blunted off to some extent, no doubt, by fusion with the surroundings. If there is no sensation at that point, the related part in the mass will be correspondingly weak. A difference of quality will generally be retained. And when the area consists of a scattering of still smaller areas, the unstimulated holes in it will be somewhat contracted by the process of overlapping fusion. And so on. It will therefore be evident that every areal sensation has its own particular, more or less complex, distribution of attributive differences.

The precise study of these matters is of greater interest to the physiologist than to the psychologist. For the primary basis of them all is undoubtedly physical. The psychical side is doubtless determined entirely by some regular dependence of sensation upon physiological process —by their parallelism, as it is called. But the process of overlapping and of resultant intensities can equally well be stated for either side. A statement of the psychical process is necessary for understanding the connexions between isolated particles of sensation and areas of it.

The physiological basis of the skin senses has been the object of intense and minute study in recent years, especially since Head and his collaborators claimed to have shown the existence in the skin of two systems of receptors —" protopathic " and " epicritic," a rougher and more primitive set as well as a finer and later supply. But this theory has been rejected by later workers in spite of the immense amount of care bestowed by all upon experiment and interpretation. The ordinary and abnormal facts of skin sensitivity seem to be reducible to (1) spotwise sensitivity of the surface of the skin to the four qualities we have enumerated ; (2) complete loss thereof upon nerve section ; (3) diffusion of heavier stimuli of pressure and temperature to neighbouring normal areas ; (4) certain peculiar couplings of spots that are revealed by nerve injuries ; (5) sensitivity to pain that is spread throughout deeper regions and that is probably, though not demonstrably, spotwise.

The theory of the multiple innervation of sensory spots that was proposed by von Frey [1] and by Boring [2] is perhaps the most interesting result of all this work. It suggests means whereby the great number of sensory spots could be supplied by a relatively small number of nerve fibres and yet provide in the central nervous system in the vast majority of cases, i.e. normally, a unique excitation for each receptive spot. The false and double localisations of stimuli that sometimes occur are therefore only special or temporary disturbances of this system of connexions on the physical side. They do not in any way alter the fact that each particle of sensation has its own inherent position, whether this happens to be " false " or not, or is indistinguishable in position from other spots not very distant from it. However complex the physiological processes underlying sensation may be—and they must be very complex, involving various types of mutual inhibition and facilitation between central excitations, as well as the simpler summation of their overlapping parts, the

[1] *Ztsch. Biol.*, 1911, **56**, 537 ; 1913, **59**, 497 ; 1914, **63**, 335 ; *Ergebn., d. Physiol.*, 1913, **13**, 96. *Skand. Arch. Physiol.*, 1913, **29**, 68.

[2] *Q. J. Experimental Physiol.*, 1916, **10**, 1 ff.

interests of pure psychology are not involved so long as the resulting sensations have all the properties that belong to them generally.

It is true that this may seem to leave a very meagre substance for the groundwork of psychology. There will be all the more interest in seeing how it complicates to form the wonderfully involved structure of the human mind.

Our psychological interest in the psychophysical arrangement of the senses seems at present to be satisfied by recognising the essentially spotwise distribution of sensitivity, that at no point is seriously disputed. For even if an area be continuously sensitive in the sense that no stimulus can be set down upon it without evoking a sensation (as may well be under certain circumstances), still sensitivity depends on nerve supply, and this must be punctate, and so sensitivity must be essentially spotwise both at periphery and brain. Only we cannot then stimulate a single spot in isolation from all others—a case to which we shall find a parallel in hearing. And apart from special details required for the economy of neural connexions in the central nervous system, the features of extent, position, and intensity of sensation seem to correspond very closely with what may be considered to be the probable result in the central nervous system (in the cortex) of the stimulation of the receptors. But until direct information regarding this resultant is obtained, our notion of it must be taken entirely by parallelism from the resultant sensations themselves. In fact, it is the very cogency of this idea of psychophysical parallelism (i.e. between the sensory datum and the underlying central bra n process) that makes the purely psychological analysis of these elementary sensations so important. The psychological side is the one about which we can get direct information, and it is important to make it as accurate as possible, so that we may win the best idea of its neural counterpart.

Certain combinations of skin sensations are of interest. Heat is the simultaneous occurrence of warmth and cold on the same part of the skin. The cold spots are excited not only by low temperatures, but also by temperatures higher than those that will arouse the warmth spots only. The cold spots react more quickly than the warm ones, so that for a brief instant cold water and hot water feel alike, e.g. when a finger or a foot is jerked through a stream of water. The test may be made more effective if the hand or foot is immersed in warm water (e.g. in a bath) into which streams of cold and hot water are running. All the warmth spots of the skin are already excited, and the effect of momentary contact with either stream of water is to rouse certain cold spots as well. It is then difficult to distinguish which stream is which, until the pain of the hot water appears. According to Cutolo [1] "Heat, a cutaneous quality that is neither warmth nor cold, may result from the simultaneous stimulation of warm and cold spots," as Alrutz [2] said. But Cutolo does not agree with Thunberg [3] that heat is a mixed sensation; he finds, rather, that heat itself mixes and fuses with warmth or cold; and that there may be spatial mixtures, and probably fusions of warmth and heat or of cold and heat at the same place. And his observers are not agreed as regards the presence of the quality of pain in the experience of heat. So here heat is a special quality of sensation, a sort of concomitant sensation probably, that has at least not yet been excited in isolation.

Wetness is a combination of temperature and pressure, while dryness is a different disposition of these senses. Apart from movement of the skin relatively to the surface of contact smoothness and roughness become evenness and unevenness. Oiliness is a blend of warmth and pressure. Complete study of these and other such blends of skin sensation involves careful observation under the conditions that naturally give rise to the "perceptions," followed by a synthesis of the effect from its immediate physiological conditions. Thus oiliness may be evoked by bending a hair with a heated cylinder without touching the skin.[4]

[1] *Amer. J. Psych.*, 1918, **29**, 442; and Alston, *ibid.*, 1920, **31**, 303.
[2] *Skand. Arch. Physiol.*, 1908, **20**, 371.
[3] Nagel's *Handbuch der Physiol. des Menschen*, 1905, **3**, 647 ff.
[4] Cobbey and Sullivan, *Amer. J. Psych.*, 1922, **33**, 121 ff.

Itching and tickling are feelings that present numerous obscurities and difficulties. Alrutz[1] after lengthy review concludes that they are variants of one and the same quality produced by different manners of stimulation. They seem to be independent of the pressure sense, but not of the sense of pain. They are marked by radiating character, strong tendency to produce reflex action (which sometimes lapses and can be suppressed), and by special "feeling-tone." But others think that tickle is due to partial activity of touch and itch to that of pain.[2]

It may be useful at this point to recount the chief physiological problems of skin-sensitivity, so that we may know them as such and recognise how much of what is usually displayed as psychology of the senses is really physiological matter. These are such as the following: (1) How is each sense distributed over the skin or throughout the body? (2) What distinguishable organs in the skin are similarly distributed? (3) What is the precise physical force to which that organ responds most easily, or what is the "adequate" stimulus? (4) How does this stimulus affect the organ when applied for a short time or for a longer time, and what are its after-effects as judged by our sensations? (5) What other forces than the adequate one will excite the organ? (6) How does the organ work? (7) Do the organs for any quality form a single homogenous system, or are there several systems, e.g. superficial and deep organs, etc? (8) By what paths in the spinal cord and brain is each organ connected with the part whose function immediately subserves sensation, and what other connexions are formed over these paths? (9) Why are sensations (especially pains) often "referred" to parts where there is at the moment no corresponding (algic) stimulus? (10) How do simultaneously excited organs affect each other's action? And so on.

It will readily be seen from the terms in which these questions are formulated that they are not in the least concerned to increase our knowledge of the nature, varieties, and properties of sensory experiences. In fact, in so far as

[1] Loc. cit.

[2] For a figure illustrating the probable affinities of the skin senses, cf. Titchener, *Amer. J. Psych.*, 1920, **31**, 212 ff.

such questions can be answered by direct experiment upon, and observation of, receptors and their attached transmittors or nerves, the physiologist may ignore the existence of sensations altogether, just as in the study of the animal organism, especially in its lower orders, he is compelled to do. In other words the physiologist is by definition a "behaviourist" and not a psychologist. The latter has an independent, though correlated, task.

CHAPTER III

THE INNER SENSES

THE senses of the first group have been called the "near" senses, though obviously the sense of warmth is as "far" as one could wish a sense to be. But we do not so much use our sense of warmth to find the place and form of warm objects as to feel the warmth they produce in ourselves, so that warmth acts almost always as a "near" sense. These senses are excited from without the body by forces more or less closely in contact with it. The variable extent of the forces and their movements over the large sensitive surface produce varying changes in the sensations and make them easy to observe and to analyse.

For the second group of senses almost the contrary is true. No sensitive spots here lie open to easy stimulation. The receptive organs are embedded in the limbs—about the muscles and joints—or in the inner surfaces of the alimentary canal and its adjuncts, etc. The nature of the forces that actually stimulate them is far from obvious, and it is difficult or impossible to control the intensity and extent of their application. Even yet there is no definite unanimity of opinion as to their location and nature, although our knowledge has steadied up in recent years towards more definite results. This is the result of the intensive study and careful experimentation to which these medically so important senses have been subjected.

The sense of weight or the muscular sense is perhaps the most clearly established. It is, of course, associated particularly with the act of weighing things or of judging force for the purposes of knowledge. Its general concern is the regulation of the innervation of muscles in relation to any conscious process. A contracting muscle must set free force enough to overcome the load it bears, namely, its own parts, the limb it is attached to, and any weight bound to the latter. In judging weights we try to abstract from the former so as to get as clear a notion as possible of the weight held by the limb. But the weight we actually feel is always the sum total. And by relieving the muscle of the weight of the limb for some time (as in a bath) it is easy to feel this whole weight vividly for an instant afterwards. It is a burden we ignore unless our muscles are unusually weak or tired.

In the act of careful weighing, all variable aspects of the muscular sensations as well as of the whole action involved, e.g. its speed, the range of the limb's movements, the expectation of weight we bring to the act, the muscles used, the manner of grasping the object, etc. (cf. p. 105), must be kept constant. Under these circumstances the weight felt varies with the relative turning force from the point of application to the joint over which the muscle acts. And as the weight of the limb itself is constant, the added weight then weighs in proportion to its distance from the joint. Thus 1 kilogram at a distance of 30 cm. from the shoulder joint will feel equal to half a kilogram at 60 cm.[1] Clearly we can expect great accuracy only when we judge equality and difference of weights, not when we try to find a weight that feels twice as heavy as another. For if the weight of the arm in the posture adopted be 160 kg. cm., the one weight felt will be $160+x$, the other $160+2x$, or e.g. ($x=30$) 190 and 220 kg. cm. Only long "experience" in estimating weight could teach us to call the latter double the former. Of the methods of estimating weight the "tossing" one is best. For the muscle is only a short time in play, fatigue is less, and the sensations to be compared are brought temporarily close together.

Of the attributes of weight intensity is by far the most important, since it alone is of considerable practical value and by it chiefly the amount of a weight is judged. The positional attribute of weight sensations doubtless differs from muscle to muscle and probably enables us to know which muscle is involved in any act of weighing or which

[1] M. v. Frey, "Studien über den Kraftsinn." *Ztsch. Biol.*, 1913, **63**, 129 ff.

muscle may have contracted involuntarily. But we hardly ever pay explicit attention to this aspect of muscular sense. For muscles do not move about in the body, and the muscular movement in which we are interested is voluntary, so that we somehow "know" beforehand which muscles we are going to move. What exactly constitutes this knowledge no one yet knows, and we can hardly guess with any prospect of success. But it seems necessary at least to postulate some difference in the sensations from different muscles, if only for the purpose of regulating such an act as weighing. And the attribute of position would yield this distinction.

The extent or mass of weight sensations seems to vary from small to large muscles and probably also to some extent in one and the same muscle as more or less of it is actually innervated in the act of lifting. But it has little practical importance for the same reasons.

A weight placed upon the palm of the hand lying on a table also gives a sensation of a certain intensity, extent, and position. But the quality of the sensation is now pressure or touch, which is noticeably different from the quality of muscular sensation. And the differences of load we can distinguish by the two senses differ considerably. They are for pressure one in forty and for weight one in seventy (von Frey, loc. cit.) But authorities differ very greatly about the exact values of such ratios.[1]

The temporal attributes of the senses generally call for so little comment that we shall postpone further notice of them until we deal with our sense of time.

A special and distinct sense associated with the relative positions (and movements) of the parts bound together in a joint has long been assumed to exist, although the location of its receptor organs had never been determined. But it has recently been shown by von Frey and O. B. Meyer, that, within the normal range of articular positions, only sensations of the skin-sense of pressure are involved in our awareness of these relative positions.

Von Frey's experiments[2] consisted in moving the

[1] Cf. Whipple, *Manual of Mental and Physical Tests*, vol. i, p. 223. Baltimore.

[2] *Ztsch. Biol.*, 1918, **68**, 301 ff.

thumb on its basal joint and the lower arm and hand on the elbow joint with very small angular accelerations and speeds. Generally a movement through ½ to 1° sufficed for the recognition of a movement and its direction.

Not only does this just noticeable difference vary in amount from person to person and from one joint to another (thumb ½°, elbow 1°), but it is also affected by the angular velocity of movement, by the initial position before movement (being slightly smaller—by ¼°—from positions of extreme flexion than from other angular positions of the elbow joint), and in general by the direction of movement (being better in great extension for more extension and in great flexion for more flexion than for the opposite directions).

Anæsthetisation of different parts of the skin shows that the sensations by which movement is detected originate partly in regions beyond the joint where the moving force is applied and partly in the region of the joint moved.

And all these sensations are pressure sensations, showing their kinship with pressure not only by direct observation, but also by their low threshold, by the certainty with which their direction of change is recognised, by their dependence on velocity (of displacement of stimulus, or of deformation of the skin), as well as by their dependence on the tension and temperature of the skin. A plaster fixed upon the skin over the elbow with its centre on the olecranon increased the sensitivity to flexion by ¼° and decreased it for extension by a somewhat similar amount. And, as every one knows, low temperature reduces the sensitivity of the skin to touch and makes our movements dull and awkward.

Von Frey failed to detect the co-operation of any other senses in the discrimination of such movements, and for various reasons deems it improbable. But on approaching the extreme limits of articular movement painful sensations appear that presumably come from the bands of the joints and from the sinew sheaths.

In a subject in whom the opposed surfaces of the elbow joint had been removed to procure the formation of a new joint, sensitivity to movement was found to be practically intact.[1]

[1] Von Frey, *ibid.*, 339 ff.

It has frequently been asserted that in cases of locomotor ataxia articular sense is lost while skin sense and muscular power remain intact. The patient can therefore control his movements so long as he is able to see their progress and effect. But when his vision is distracted, as when he looks up at a clock when walking hurriedly or running, he will probably lose his balance and fall. It is usually under such circumstances that he first becomes aware of his disability. But in the tests applied to such cases hitherto—flexion of the lower upon the upper arm by a physician grasping both—sufficient care was not taken to see that no change of skin tension spread to the intact areas at the shoulder. And von Frey proved on himself that during anæsthesia of the wrist and elbow joints, when the skin round the wrist was completely, and that of the lower arm for the most part, insensitive, he could neither hold a dish tolerably level, nor put a fork into his mouth, nor touch his eye with his finger, without the use and control of vision.

Faradisation of the hand that takes part in a movement at the elbow lowers the threshold of movement distinctly, whereas faradisation of the other hand does not. Von Frey's experiments on this point prove that sensations from the skin of the hand are important even in movements of the forearm in a horizontal plane. Faradisation at the elbow end also reduces the threshold to about the same degree. But when a muscle is stimulated electrically, we do not feel any movement unless one is actually taking place.

Jointless organs like the tongue, even though they are well supplied with pressure and muscle sense, seem to have a poor sense of position. The reason probably is that, being devoid of bony frames, their surface tensions and pressures are not nearly so regularly and delicately affected by their change of posture.

The functions of articular sense are so important in many connexions that it is useful to consider them as a special sense in spite of von Frey's reduction of them to pressure sensations. In fact, this sort of distinction is already familiar in their older name of " active touch " as against the passive touch exerted by external objects.

And besides we must carefully consider how these "active" pressure-sensations fulfil the functions that have been familiar to us as articular. We shall therefore continue to to use the expression articular sense or articular pressure as distinct from skin pressure for those sensations of pressure that are evoked by movements of the joints and that we apprehend as the relative positions or movements of the parts of these joints.

Of the attributes we can see in articular sensations only one quality—now "pressure." Variations of intensity seem to be hardly present, unless it be in the progress towards disappearance of the sense in resting adaptation. The attribute of extent would appear in the more massive feelings associated with the posture of large limbs as compared with small ones, and would simply be due to the larger areas of skin affected by the changing tensions about large joints. In contrast with muscular sensation the all-important variant of articular sense is "position," either as given singly, or serially in movements. The only important question therefore is: how are the varying positions and unvarying intensities of articular sense related to the probably varying intensities of pressure-sensations whose "positions" no doubt also change from moment to moment on movement of the joint? Varying tensions of skin must produce varying intensities of pressure sense at often different points of the whole skin area affected by a joint.

This is a matter upon which we need a good deal more enlightenment by experimental means. But there is this advantage in the analysis into pressure-sensations that it is now easier to see how the position of any touch spot, e.g. a spot on the tip of an exploring finger, is altered if the altering circumstances already lie within the field of touch than if they belonged to quite a different sense, a sense of articular quality. We must not suppose that the articular pressures are absorbed into the sensation of touch on the finger tip and lost in its altered aspect of position. The spot on the finger tip is changed in itself as little as they are: but together they devise for the spot on the finger tip a new spatial localisation. And that is usually the object of our practical attention. We have no practical concern with analysis into elementary components. If we had, we should not have required to discover articular pressures now. We shall consider the question of spatial localisation more fully later on.

A distinction has sometimes been made between sensations of position and sensations of movement of the joints. In fact, separate senses have been postulated for them. We shall consider the experience of motion later by itself. But if we do not feel the need for a sense of moving touch as well as for a sense of passive pressure, we shall hardly find it necessary to posit these two senses now. We naturally tend to suppose that a moving touch includes, or simply consists of, the series of touch particles we get if we separately stimulate every pressure spot that the moving stimulus traverses. The only difference is that in motion the whole series occurs in a continuous streak. Similarly in vision. In articular work some prejudice is raised by the critical idea that we ought therefore to judge the extent of a movement by noticing first the position at the beginning of the movement and then the one at the end of it, and by inferring the extent of the movement from them. This criticism is as wrong as it would be if it were applied to touch or vision. Nor should we have to be aware of every position the motion passed through, as a definite separate state. For that would imply that successive "spots" of sensation are always separated by a distinct gap of no sensation or of felt distance between them, which is not so. The distance involved between spots is a distance between the points of the skin most sensitive to the appropriate stimulus. So there can be no harm in saying that an articular movement consists of all the articular positions the motion passes through. Each of these would be felt as an articular position if it were given separately without change. But in a motion it is not so given. And yet the first and last positions as well as the intervening series and also the rate and extent of the movement are all open to observation according to the disposition of the attention at the moment.

Nevertheless, we soon lose all feeling of articular position if we carefully rest a limb. If the attention is thoroughly diverted during a movement of the arm, we remain unaware of the final position for a time, just as we do in general after waking peacefully from sleep. In both cases feeling is restored at once on the slightest movement. These seem to be the natural facts of adaptation, familiar in passive pressure and in vision, especially peripheral vision. So we also readily feel the motions of parts of our toes, although we should be hard put to it to guess their relative positions when they are at rest. In parts that are frequently seen and delicately moved, such as the upper arm, the forearm, and the fingers, we have a steady feeling for position as well as a keen sense of motion. Our conscious purposes oftener involve their use and therefore we learn to observe them better. They form important data upon which we construct our spatial world. The blind, owing to their greater practice and dependence on this sense, have a finer discrimination in its use.

Judgments of the extent of a movement are very much affected by the speed with which the movement is carried out and the time the movement takes. In fact, if a constant speed is adopted, the duration of movements (especially such as are made in different regions of the available joint motion) may be judged instead of the inherent extent of it, so that times being equal, extents will be declared equal, and times being longer or shorter, extents will be overestimated and underestimated. Experimental results are not quite decisive as to the degree to which the judgment of extent is influenced by the judgment of speed and the time of movement. And this ambiguity is perhaps related to the nature of judgments of speed-time. Clearly a judgment of mere time spent could not control an extent apart from some control of speed. And speed implies appreciation of the extent passed over in the unit of time. It is or contains these two things (extent and time) indissolubly within it. Speed, however, as we shall see, can be judged by itself, apart from any analysis of it into its original components, extent and time. So while speed-time may be a convenient and sometimes easier method of gauging extent, we are able to gauge extent, not only in this synthesis indirectly, but for itself apart from time. The most frequent or most convenient means of judgment does not always point to the primary basis of judgment, an important truth we find exemplified in all sorts of mental processes. Long practice, however, seems here to eliminate the speed-habit of judgment in favour of judgments of extent.

Labyrinthine senses.—The organ of hearing is embedded in a complex, irregularly shaped cavity towards which the opening of the external ear leads, known as the labyrinth. The cochlear part of it is exclusively devoted to the functions of hearing. But in the other parts—the three semicircular canals and the utricle and saccule, there are five sets of receptors which are associated with sensations of movement and of posture of the body (*quâ* head) as a whole.

The theory of the semicircular organs is simple and well established. Rotation of the head causes the lymph in these tubes to move under its own inertia through them in a direction opposite to that of the motion of the head. In other words, when the head moves, so does the tube ; but the fluid (like the tea in a cup that is turned round on its saucer) lags behind, and so moves over the projecting hairs of the receptor area in a certain direction. If rotation continues at an even rate, the friction between the tube wall and the lymph will gradually cause both to move without any motion relatively to one another. Thereafter on stoppage of rotation the lymph will move on under its momentum, thus moving within the tube in the direction opposed to that produced when movement of the head first began.

Our sensations normally correspond to these physical differences. At first on passive rotation on a swivel-chair or turn-table we feel motion in one direction ; gradually this fades out, if there is no acceleration of the physical movement ; on stoppage we feel a sudden motion in the opposite direction, which in turn gradually fades out. The same holds for rectilinear movements.

These sensations can easily be shown to depend upon some organ in the head ; for any alteration in the posture of the head at the stoppage of motion changes the plane of the "illusory" motion correspondingly. The head, of course, carries the relative motion, once set up, unalterably with it, as the eye carries an after image when it moves. And movement of the lymph in the canal of a living pigeon has been actually observed microscopically.[1]

When the body lies relaxed upon a turn-table the "illusory" after-motion is indistinguishable from the first "real" motion, especially if vision has been excluded. If the illusory motion is produced by rotation on the heel or the like, the after effect is *obviously* illusory, as it is inconsistent with the presentations of vision. This state of conflict is highly disconcerting, being the most acute state of giddiness. It is greatly heightened by the "nystagmus" of the eyes that is reflexly produced by the normal stimulation of the semicircular receptors. The eyes (as if they were fixating a point outside of us) are moved gradually in the direction opposed to the rotation of the head (or "in the direction of the endolymph movement") and quickly jerked back again (as if to fixate a new point outside of us as we turn). In the after-effect all this is, of course, useless and confusing. It is what then seems to make the room turn round.

When rotation is begun imperceptibly (first rotation in some twenty seconds) and very slowly increased, the subject, whose eyes are closed, becomes aware of rotation after about half a rotation, then somewhere between the first and the tenth rotation, while still accelerating, rotation seems to decrease, stop, and then suddenly reverse. This reversal gradually disappears before the maximum rotation (120° to 180° per sec.) is reached. Then on slow and gradual deceleration, the ordinary illusion of reversed rotation appears, gradually reaches a maximum and dies out. Six to ten seconds after stopping a "positive after-image" of rotation appears, similarly increasing to a maximum and then fading away. This may be followed by a faint "negative after-image" of rotation (i.e. in the opposite direction). The reversal of direction during acceleration and these after-images while the subject is at rest, seem difficult to explain on the theory just stated. They suggest the existence of a central

[1] Maier and Lion, *Arch. ges. Physiol.*, 1921, **187**, 47 ff.

compensating factor, some antagonistic force that tends to inhibit the primary sensory effects of a process long continued.[1]

Giddiness thus seems to be the acute inco-ordination of sensory presentations from different senses (here vision and muscular-articular kinæsthesis as well as changes of pressure due to rotation and its cessation). It arises in less acute forms on other similar occasions, as when we sit in a train looking at another train that has just begun to move; or in the after-effect of seen movement (cf. p. 116); or on looking down from heights (or sometimes up to heights) where we lose touch with our visual apprehension of the ground we stand on, that is normally closely co-ordinated with our muscular-articular sense of posture on the ground. Fit and practised people are immune to these occasions of giddiness, while to prevent it others prepare themselves by getting a keener sense of their limbs for the time being or by giving the leg some extra contact. Some men become giddy more easily then others, e.g. in the work of aviation. As children they could not swing with pleasure and some of them were habitually sick in the train. This is not a pathological condition, but a lack of such full control of impulses originating in the semicircular canals as is found in most healthy individuals. And when control is acquired it can be disturbed by suitable distracting conditions of appropriate force, just as every man (with normal organs) can be made giddy by sufficiently intense rotation. Other forms of inco-ordination may cause some momentary giddiness, e.g. sudden loss of orientation, or of memory, or the mental paralysis of sudden confusion, shock, etc. A person in such condition may stumble and reel as if mildly intoxicated.

The ampular organs are also connected reflexly with the body musculature. Such mechanisms are of the greatest importance in the act of balancing, especially after sudden disturbances of balance. We should have no time to recover if the action were solely under the control of our sensations and will. A beautiful example of this reflex change of posture can be got from the cat, if it is nursed into repose on its back in the palms of one's hands and

[1] Cf. R. Dodge, *J. Exper. Ps.*, 1923, 6, 1 ff.

then suddenly let fall. It will turn round within a very short distance so as to land evenly on its feet. Similarly a child falling forwards throws up its arms and pulls back its head. Of course in an active conscious animal that may fall or lose balance in any sort of posture and may need to grab at some support while falling the process of balancing must be under control, even though reflexly initiated and supported, just as the process of walking is. And so we find it in the usual tests for normal labyrinthine action of pointing (or " past pointing "). The subject is asked to point at an object on the cessation of rotation and does so, allowing for his experience of movement, i.e. he points past the object in a direction contrary to that in which he feels he is moving. So in the reaction to the feeling of motion after rotation we control the body to suit this feeling, but really wrongly, and so fall in the direction opposed to this feeling. In other words, we throw ourselves down, it may be (not voluntarily, of course) just as we violently throw ourselves forwards when our heels slip forwards and the body backwards. There is also a disturbance in the localisation of sounds, which may similarly be explained, rather than by any direct action of rotation upon the special organs of hearing.

Thus we have reason to suspect that the motion we feel on rotation is visual and muscular-articular motion. And the question arises whether we get any sense of motion at all directly and exclusively from the semicircular receptors. This doubt is strengthened by several lines of evidence : (1) that no nerve fibres connect these receptors with the cerebral cortex. " The fibres conveying the impulses producing vertigo go through the cerebellum *en route* for the cerebrum," [1] and (2) there is evidence that voluntary inhibition of nystagmus does away with the sense of bodily rotation, not merely after the rotation has stopped, but during the actual rotation also. This explains the fact that whereas the novice regularly suffers from rotary giddiness after waltzing, practice very soon dispels the last trace of any such thing. Rotary giddiness

[1] J. H. Jones, *Equilibrium and Stability*, 1918, p. 123. According to Magnus and de Kleijn the medulla and mid-brain is the central seat of the labyrinth reflexes in cats and rabbits.

on other occasions is controlled by special acts of vision and fixation of eyes and by body control. As the head in ordinary activities is constantly being turned and accelerated, such control must be continuously exercised and may occasionally lapse more or less, as in certain disturbances of digestion, etc. (3) Apparent feelings of motion of the body as a whole, as in a train that is moving without acceleration, are often purely visual or " inferred," though difficult to remove. But on shutting the eyes for a time we notice that we can equally readily imagine that we are moving forwards or backwards or are merely being " dirled " without any such motion. We should, therefore, be impelled to infer that there is no special and proper ampullar sense of motion, however receptive the ampullar organs may be to the stimulus of (acceleration of) rotary or rectilinear movement.

The receptor organs of the utricle and saccule are associated with our sense of the position of the body as a whole, especially in its orientation to the vertical. In animals such as frogs, etc., these organs determine the upright posture; and, if iron-filings be substituted (at the change of carapace) for the grains of sand that in some of them load the hairs of the organs, pulling the latter aside and so stimulating them on change of posture, the creature may by suitable magnetic action be made to turn over on to its back and stay there. Similarly a cyclist turning a corner feels himself to be upright even though he is actually inclined at a considerable angle to the ground. Gravity and centrifugal force give these receptors the stimulus usual during the upright posture. If a person on being thus turned tries to put a stick into the vertical position he does so true to his momentary sense of the vertical and not to the physical-vertical. Of course, if the body did not thus adjust itself, it would fall over in the direction of its motion before turning, as a runaway tram-car does at a turning. Thus the body's muscular-articular sense of balance must be involved in the action. It has been said that persons immersed in deep water while bathing run the risk of drowning by want of a proper sense of direction, if these organs are so abnormal that they are incapable of rotary giddiness. But this statement has recently been denied.[1] Such persons under ordinary circumstances are quite well aware of their relation to the vertical. And we seem to have as good a sense of the inclination of the body when the head is fixed as conversely. Hence that we actually get sensation directly from these receptors is perhaps more doubtful than in the case of the ampullar organs.

The interoceptive senses are limited to small areas of the alimentary tract and its adjuncts. Hunger and thirst are familiar and distinctive examples. Hunger is excited by the rhythmical contractions of the walls of the stomach and perhaps also of the œsophagus. It contains an element of dull pain and is otherwise perhaps more like the sense of muscular strain or weight than any other. Thirst is excited by dryness of the mouth and pharynx. And its psychological quality seems accordingly to be simply dryness of a special " position." We must therefore have to learn to know it or to act towards it as thirst. These and other " organic " sensations (e.g. those connected with evacuation of the rectum and bladder and the feeling of nausea) are of little importance for knowledge. They are of some importance in the study of emotion, which by one theory is said to consist of the sensations evoked reflexly from our viscera and other internal parts by various objects (the objects of our emotion). They generally take the form of vaguely defined lumps or masses of pain and pressure, which we locate on the whole with fair accuracy near the parts where their organs probably lie. Distinct form would be wasted upon them, because their practically important aspects are merely (the time of) their occurrence and their intensity. There is no need for us to notice where we feel hungry nor how big our hunger is. And yet hunger is undoubtedly a big feeling made up, like all other big sensations, of a large number of little bits (or " particles ") of hunger, each one excited from a single receptive organ attached to an afferent nerve. Hunger at its climax is surely much bigger as well as more intense than the first twinge of it.

The important condition of appetite does not seem to be

[1] K. Beck, *Ztsch. Sinnesphys.*, 1912, **46**, 362 ff.

a primitive sensation so much as an attitude towards foods based on our memory of their taste and smell, excited by the sight or smell of them, and usually heightened by the actual taste of them. It is the " urge-towards-more-of-that " feeling, presumably implying interadjustment of stimulus and organism on the basis of habit, reinforced it may be by higher mental processes of knowledge. Carlson,[1] however, considers appetite to be a special stomachic sense, distinct from hunger.

The sexual sensation, which we may call lust, may be noticed at this point as a special sense. It seems to be rather a skin sense than an " organic " sense and to share the punctate and other characteristics of skin senses.[2]

[1] A. J. Carlson, *The Control of Hunger in Health and Disease.* Chicago, 1916.

[2] S. Baglioni, *Arch. ges. Phys.*, 1913, **159**, 361 ff.

CHAPTER IV

THE HIGHER SENSES—HEARING

SOUNDS fall obviously into two classes—noises and tones. Both occur in great variety, and the question at once arises what is the relation between them. The general tendency hitherto has been to regard the noises as really consisting of a great many tones. For there are far many more kinds of noise than of tone. It is very difficult to suggest any scheme or arrangement which will give every kind of noise its proper place, but for any kind of instrument the tones it produces clearly form a regular series. Compared together the series from different instruments are partly the same, partly different; for while we can play the same melody on many instruments —violin, voice, or piano, we can still recognise the instrument used by the kind of tone it produces. Thus our first special problem is to show the relation between the different series of instrumental tones.

By simple experiment we can find that an instrumental tone is not as simple as it seems, but really consists of a small group or blend of tones. These are called partials of the whole instrumental tone. In all tones of the same pitch from different instruments there is an identical component, called the "fundamental." It is the lowest in pitch of all the partials of the tone. It is this lowest component that gives the whole blend an apparent pitch. In every instrumental tone the fundamental is accompanied by various other higher components, called upper partials. These commonly bear a certain relation to the fundamental that is determined by the physical vibrations of the instrument used. When an instrument is intentionally brought into one rate of vibration, as when you strike a certain note on the piano or sing a certain pitch, it falls at the same time into other rates of vibration that are simple multiples of the rate intended. The pitches of the partials vary accordingly. The complete series of the simple multiples gives the following relative pitches for each partial, if we suppose for example that the fundamental bears the musical name " c " or " f."

Rel. rates of vib.	1	2	3	4	5	6	7	8	9	10	etc.
Relative pitch	c	c^1	g^1	c^2	e^2	g^2	$<b^{b2}$	c^3	d^3	e^3	etc.
	f	f^1	c^2	f^2	a^2	c^3	$<e^{b3}$	f^3	g^3	a^3	etc.
Partial No.	1	2	3	4	5	6	7	8	9	10	etc.

The partials of the complete series may easily be found for any other fundamental by transposing the whole series by the same interval as is required to turn "c" or "f" into the pitch of the given fundamental.

The group of partials that accompanies the fundamental differs from instrument to instrument and is a selection from this complete series. Tuning forks and flutes have very few partials, the piano has the first six or seven, trumpet tones have many high partials, etc. The relative intensity of the partials that are present also varies from instrument to instrument and the manner of action of the instrument from moment to moment also modifies the partials of its tones.

By this analysis we see that all varieties of instrumental tones are merely assortments of the pure tones of a single series, duly subordinated in intensity to their fundamental, which determines the pitch of the whole, and which seems merely to change its hue or blend by the admixture of the different sets of partials. A good singer or violin player can make the blend of the tone he produces change considerably without altering the (fundamental) pitch of the tone in the least. This is done by setting the vocal organs (including the mouth, etc.) differently or by bowing the string at a different point of its length, and is one of the great charms of musical variety.

A pure tone therefore contains only one appreciable pitch. The lowest audible tone corresponds to about 16 vibrations of the air per second, the highest to 20,000 or more. The series of pure tones stretches continuously between these limits, and every pure tone as well as every ordinary instrumental tone in respect of its nominal or fundamental pitch occupies a certain position in the series.

As tones have thus been reduced to a relatively small and definite number, we naturally expect to be able to reduce noises to the same components. For noises in many ways seem to be only complex and rough tones. Many tones of neighbouring pitch sounded together make a noisier effect than does a smaller or musical group of tones. And in noises various partials may be detected by the same sort of analysis as is used for musical tones. Physical and mathematical theory also sees in the vibrations of the air that correspond to noise only a very complex system of the vibrations that correspond to pure tones. Up to a point the reduction of noise to tones is quite a proper idea, but we require to pursue the psychological analysis of tones somewhat further before we can state the relation between them exactly. Tone does not seem to be the pure quality incapable of further analysis that it is commonly supposed to be when it is taken for the element to which all sorts of sounds are to be reduced. It seems itself to be complex, and so capable of analysis into parts, which may also be the parts that make up noises.

A tone is rather a mass or extent of sound, comparable with the mass of warmth got from a small area of the skin. Low tones seem much bigger than high ones. In fact, the extent, or as it is commonly termed, the volume [1] of tones decreases as the pitch rises. We can represent this size by a line, so that we may draw a long line for a low tone and a short line for a high tone; we may also suppose that as a large extent of warmth consists of all the particles of warmth provided by the area warmed, so a large tone consists really of a great number of sound particles each possessing its own definite " position " among the rest.

All tones have the further characteristic of smoothness and regularity. We therefore have all the data required for the application of Bernstein's theory of the " spot " of sensation to tone. We have only to add that the pitch of a tone will clearly be that point of its extent that is most

[1] The meaning of this term should not be confused with its popular use as a name for the intensity of sound.

intense. The most likely position for this prominent point in a smoothly graded mass is the centre of it. So the diagram of any tone, larger or smaller in the scale according to its mass, would be thus:

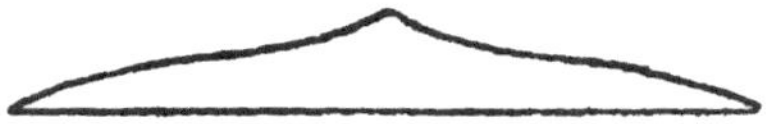

FIG. 1.[1]

But though in any one tone only one sound-particle is strongly marked as to position, yet, as we plainly hear in the next noticeably higher or lower tone the next sound particle along the line in either direction is predominant. For the pitch has shifted up or down, i.e. one place along in the direction we call by metaphor "up" or "down." So we can bring all tones together into one figure (Fig. 2).

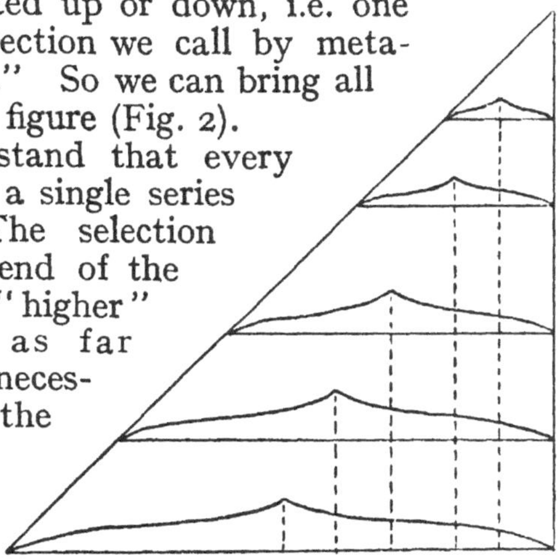

FIG. 2.

We now can understand that every tone consists of part of a single series of sound-particles. The selection always begins at the end of the series that we call the "higher" end, and proceeds as far "downwards" as is necessary to make up the size of tone required. The lowest audible tone contains twice as many sound-particles as the whole series of

[1] Bernstein's figure is usually represented as a little mound, showing from above no concavity. The intensive outline of tone displayed above is chosen on the grounds advanced in my *Psychology of Sound*, p. 164. It might also be derived from the spread of resonance on the basilar membrane, from the chief point of resonance outwards in opposite directions: towards apex and basis of the cochlea, in order to agree with Wilkinson and Gray's theory of the action of the cochlea. But we do not know yet what the course and scope of this range of resonance is. Our aim here is to depict the relations between tones systematically. And as long as there is a continuous decrease from a maximum intensity to nil on either side, our picture will not be affected by minor differences such as these which must for some time remain matters of speculation.

4

pitches actually reveals to us one by one in just noticeably different tones. The lower half of the whole series of sound-particles can evidently never be heard as pitches.

Now it is easy to see what noises are. There are, of course, blends of noises as well as of tones. And partial noises or tones can be found in some noises. But some noises defy any proper analysis by ear. These and any residual noises are rough and irregular sounds, containing either no detectable pitch or only a more or less indefinite one, discernible after some comparison. Their mass is generally more readily distinguished than their pitch. They are irregularly graded masses of sound, in which no one pitch stands out clearly amongst the sound-particles of which they consist. Noises and tones are both reducible to the same series of sound-particles. The difference is comparable to that between smooth and rough pressure contacts.

Persons who can distinguish very small differences between tones and perhaps sing them accurately are said to have a good ear. But others can hardly distinguish tones that differ by a semitone, or a tone, or even more. We may suppose that their ears are of too rough a texture in some essential part to give the regular grading of mass that tone requires. So the pitch point of tones is then more or less obliterated. That will not prevent them hearing either noises or tones as some sort of sounds and of distinguishing them from one another too, either by their intensive grading or at least by their mass. But tones will be heard in a roughened form as a kind of noise, the least disagreeable kind of noise, as unmusical persons sometimes say. The relations between tones that make music must then be obscured almost as much as they are for us in very noisy tones or in very " ragged " orchestral playing. We can therefore understand why they learn to recognise noises, e.g. the so important noises of speech ; they may even be able to learn them as readily as do people whose ears are tonal, but it is not very likely. Those who learn to notice, remember, and name tones and their groupings with exceptional ease probably have ears of a finer texture than usual. Most people readily distinguish a difference of from one to three vibrations per second. From there the frequency falls off rapidly into a slowly decreasing tail that reaches beyond a difference of 30 vbs. per sec. (for a standard of 435 vbs.). The finest sensibility is about one-third of a vibration per sec. Of course the musical nature of the latter must be greatly heightened by the potencies of interests, training, and memory, while the opposite extreme will be exaggerated by their impotence.

Speech consists of sounds, of which the vowels are much more tonal than the consonants. No one who can hear, be his ear tonal in its texture or not, fails to distinguish them from one another. The human voice contains a great number of partials, even up to the 36th, more than five octaves above the fundamental voice pitch. These all belong to the harmonic series, being whole multiples of the vibratory rate of the fundamental. Now any element (or partial) of a vowel sound that helps to give it its peculiar character (by which we recognise it) belongs to a certain range of pitch. But it is also a partial of the voice-tone. It must therefore be that partial of the voice-tone that happens to fall within the said range of pitch, no natter what partial of the voice-sound this may be. For the range c^0 to g^{b1}, which includes the fundamental tones of human speech, the characteristic vowel ranges remain constant and lie within the ranges that are found to be characteristic of whispered vowels. When vowels are sung on a high pitch, e.g. at c^2, their differences are not so apparent; for the components of different vowels then grow more alike. Individual differences of voice, of course, alter the number of partials available for vowel production, as the analysis of instrumental tones has already shown. In men's voices I is usually rather low, somewhat resembling the vowel E. Obliteration of the high components darkens or obscures the vowel; loss of the much weaker low components brightens it.

The chief components of certain vowels are shown in Fig. 2a, taken from the work of Stumpf. The dark vowels U and O have the smaller number of partials. E and I have two maxima, E's lower one being identical with Ŏ's, I's with Ŭ's. But for some shortening of the range below for U and some raising of the range for O this Table holds for whispered vowels also. The starred points are to be considered only as the centres of a characteristic region.

Similar results were got by Helmholtz some fifty years ago, and by Miller [1] recently, all by careful experimental means. The results may be considered well established. In the Table it is noticeable that the chief components of O and A lie an octave apart, while that of U can lie an

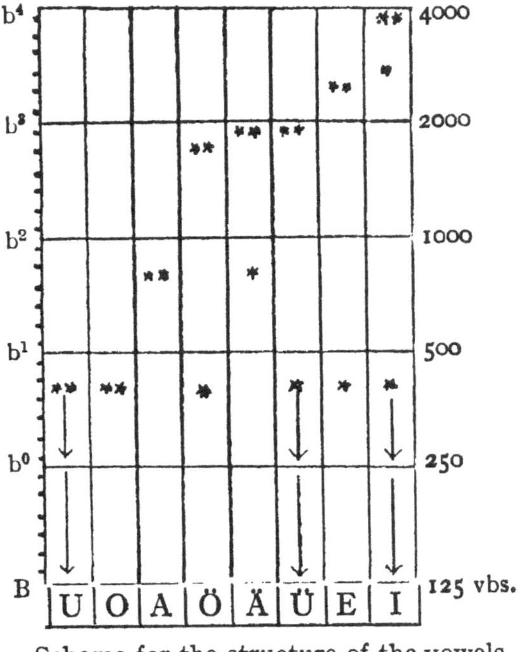

FIG. 2a.—Scheme for the structure of the vowels. The 6 notches in each octave, e.g. between b^1 and b^2, stand for c, d, e, g^b, a^b, b^b, read upwards.

octave lower. The chief components of (1)Ö (which, when the lips are opened, is a vowel on the A side of Ä); (2) of Ä (which can vary from a half-A-half-E sound to a pure E sound); and (3) of E lie an octave to an octave and fifth higher. That of I lies a little over two octaves higher. This resembles the results claimed on experimental grounds by König, Köhler,[2] and Jaensch,[3] according to whom the vowels U, O, A, E, I, stand an octave apart respectively,

[1] C. D. Miller, *The Science of Musical Sounds*. New York, 1916.

[2] *Ztsch. Psych.*, 1910, **54**, 241 ff.; 1911, **58**, 59 ff.; 1913, **64**, 92 ff.

[3] *Ztsch. Sinnesphys.*, 1913, **47**, 219 ff.

beginning with U about 250 vbs. per sec. Köhler and Jaensch add m̊ an octave below U, and the sounds s and f one and two octaves above I. No lower components were detected by these three workers.

Stumpf's vowels are, of course, German vowels, presumably with the Berlin characteristics, Ä there being much more like E than elsewhere. Miller's (U.S.A.) O sound in top is nearly the same as our English A in harp (Italian A). The frequent difficulty of making a pure I sound has already been noted. These considerations help us to bring the

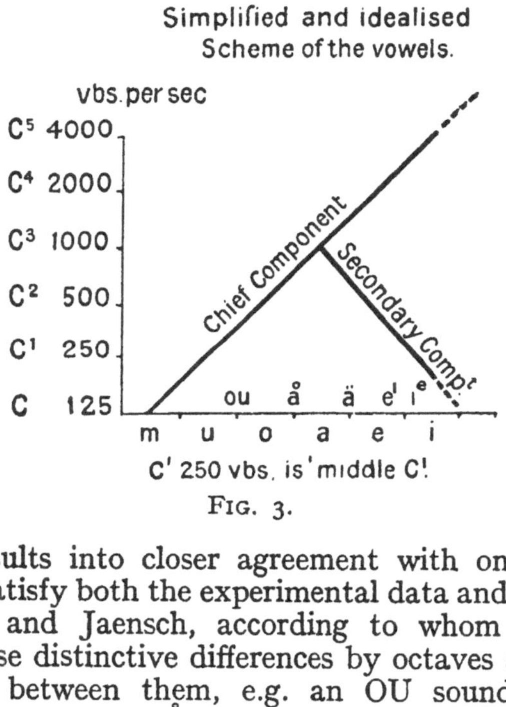

FIG. 3.

various results into closer agreement with one another, and so to satisfy both the experimental data and the claims of Köhler and Jaensch, according to whom there are besides these distinctive differences by octaves all sorts of gradations between them, e.g. an OU sound half-way between U and O, an Å (all) half-way between O and Ă (cf. the u of "but"), an Ä between A and E and many grades between E and I (bait, bit, bit in Scotch pronunciation), beat, beach.

Thus an idealised scheme of vowels might show the chief components of the series—M̊, U, O, A, E, I,—rising in octaves from 125 vibrations per second with a secondary component descending in octaves from about 1000 vbs.

This scheme certainly meets a very large proportion of the facts claimed by different workers and is easily remembered.

Semi-vowels and consonants find a similar explanation. In Table 1 the ranges of the voiceless consonants, as determined by Stumpf, are shown. Besides these peculiarities of pitch, consonants must have other characteristics to mark them off from one another, e.g. differences of distribution of intensity and also low components. The voiced nasal sounds Ng, M, N, have strong components in the upper c^3 and lower c^4 octaves. A nasal character requires a gap in the c^2 octave between the higher and lower component partials of the sound. Voiced L is reckoned to the vowels and perhaps most closely resembles the U.

The " formant " of the most important of all the vowels (A) lies at 800 vbs. From 600 to 1200 vbs. includes the most sensitive region of speech pitches. From 500 to 2100 vbs. constitues the full, necessary, and sufficient range (250 vbs. = *circa* c^1). These facts are of importance for the technique of the telephone.

TABLE 1. VOICELESS CONSONANTS.

Ch palatal	e^{b4}—d^{b5}
F	d^{b4}—d^{b5}
S	d^{b4}—c^5
L	c^4—f^4
Ng. M. N.	b^{b3}—f^4
Sh	f^3—e^{b4}
H	e^{b3}—d^{b4}
Ch guttural	d^3—a^3
K (P.T.)	d^{b3}—e^{b3}
R (lingual)	a^2—e^3

CHAPTER V

THE HIGHER SENSES—VISION, SMELL AND TASTE

AS far as the systemic attributes are concerned, vision closely resembles the skin senses, except that it is much finer and more detailed. It differs most in the vast number of its kinds or qualities. These (including the white-grey-black series) are set out diagrammatically in the colour figure on the principle of their resemblance to one another. Such an array, however, does not imply that "quality is an orderly attribute," [1] but only that it can be attached conceptually in its variations to an ordinal scheme of three dimensions.

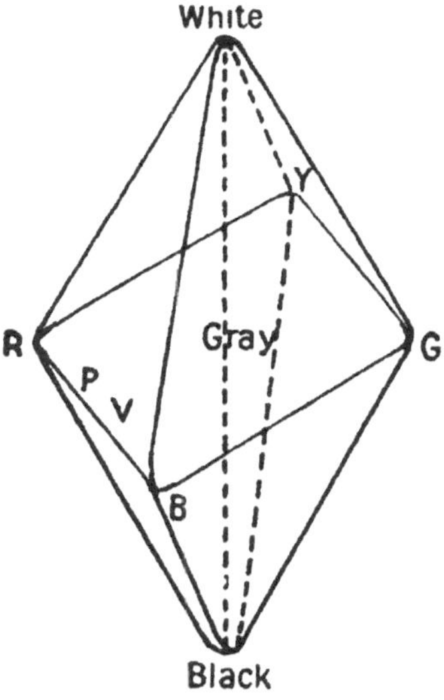

FIG. 4.

It will be noticed, for instance, that there is a continuous transition from red to yellow; colours of all degrees of resemblance to red, passing gradually through orange to yellow, can be got by the simple device of mixing different amounts of red and yellow on a rotating disc. Such mixture is the simultaneous or rapidly successive stimulation of the same part of the sensitive surface of the eye by lights of different kinds (wave-lengths), and must be distinguished from the colour changes produced by the mixture of pigments.

[1] As Lufkin asserts against me, *Amer. J. Psych.*, 1922, **33**, 128, I did not think anyone would suggest that we carry about the colour pyramid consciously or unconsciously in our minds as a sort of non-spatial colour field.

As we pass from red to the point "grey," in the middle of the figure, we see that the red, while remaining the same kind of red, fades gradually out, its place being taken up more and more by grey. This is known as the decrease of saturation of colours. The most saturated colours thus lie round the outside thick part of the figure. Colours that lie at opposite ends of any line running through the central white-grey-black line are said to be complementaries, because when mixed (e.g. by rotation) in suitable proportions, they both disappear, leaving only a grey (of the brightness which grey has at the point where the line joining the two colours in the colour figure cuts the white-grey-black line).

The darkest colour of all is black, while white is the brightest. The brightness of the other colours may be estimated by finding the height (from black) of their place in the figure: thus blue is much darker than yellow, and red is somewhat brighter than green. This brightness is a variant of sight familiar to every one, and it is commonly brought into close connexion with the idea of the intensity of light. But if we try for a moment to draw a distinction between the quality and the brightness of colour, we shall see how extremely difficult it is to do so. We cannot separate the quality of yellow from its brightness, any more than we can in the case of blue. And black and white seem to be as different in quality as red and green. In fact, it is easy to persuade oneself that by brightness we mean no more than the resemblance of any colour to black or to white. Then the whole colour-figure becomes merely a system of qualitative differences. And brightness becomes merely a kind or trend of qualitative difference, not a different sort of attribute from quality. There are many different species of quality in sensation. And qualities are often so blended together as to seem indissoluble.

This is the special anomaly of vision. Not only is it peculiar in having such a range of qualities, but it seems also to be almost devoid of any intensive changes. When we increase or decrease the intensity of physical light, the colour we see does not remain the same in quality: it always changes, growing either whiter or darker, and thus losing saturation. In fact, it is a much debated problem whether vision shows any change of intensity at all. But, of course, want of change of intensity does not necessarily imply absence of intensity altogether. And it should be possible for careful investigation to reveal at least some very slight variations of intensity in ordinary daylight vision, as in the similar case of articular sense. At the extremes in the darkest blacks (to be obtained only with the help of contrast) and in the brightest whites there are probably considerable changes of intensity, especially in the latter.

The problem of the many different qualities is solved primarily on a physiological basis. The most probable solution (of the type of Hering's) begins by the differentiation of three pairs of senses making up all colour vision, namely, white-black sense, yellow-blue sense, and red-green sense. As we should expect, these are the colours that we ordinarily tend to consider primary, unless our choice is determined chiefly by reference to the mixture of pigments. They are the greatest colour differences that occur. The members of each pair are antagonistic to one another; their colours correspond to opposite phases or directions of the same process along with a certain amount of the white-process in the case of the "positive" colours. When appropriate amounts of these opposites are mixed they cancel out and leave over this white-valency. This is the mixture of complementaries.

Thus we find that when a person is blind to either red or green he is invariably blind also to the other colour of the pair. And blindness to yellow-blue as well occurs, in an "acquired" form alone, as well as with red-green blindness in total colour blindness. About 4 per cent of white men are red-green colour blind. The proportion in other races is often much greater. This blindness seems to follow Mendel's law, being a sex-linked unit character, dominant in the male and recessive in the female, so that only few white women (*circa* 0·5 per cent) show any sign of it.[1] Probably red-green blindness, in which no other

[1] The symbols for the permutations of inheritance would therefore be: OO-OX (both normal), OO-ΘX (father colour-blind), ΘΘ-OX (mother colour-blind), (4) OΘ-ΘX or OΘ-OX (mothers tainted), and ΘΘ-ΘX (both colour-blind). No. 4 would give progeny: OΘ, ΘΘ, OX, ΘX, proportionately, and the others similarly by permutation of their symbols.

colours than yellow and blue are visible (i.e. dichromacy), is the extreme form of a weakness of red-green vision, to which an unsaturated blue-green or green appears identical with an unsaturated blue-red or red. All gradations of this weakness would therefore occur.

The retina of the normal eye is also blind round its outer edge to all colours, to red-green in a middle ring, and to no colours only in its central portion. This can easily be tested by fixating the eye on a spot and then bringing coloured objects gradually into the field of vision from its farther reaches towards the middle. The colour of purple will then be seen to change from black through blue to purple. Similar relations of colour vision hold for the passage from the normal retina into the blind spot as for the passage towards the periphery.

When the eye has steadily fixated a patch of colour for some thirty seconds and then turns to gaze upon a point on a white surface, the colour complementary to the first soon appears, coming and going gradually for almost a minute. This effect is known as the negative after-image. When a patch of grey is laid on a coloured background, we get what is called colour-contrast: the patch is changed towards the colour complementary to the background. These observations hold not only for grey and white surfaces, but for all colours. The colour looked at in the after-image is always altered by the mixture with it of the complementary of the colour previously fixated; and each colour changes any one next to it by the admixture of its own complementary and is changed by the admixture of the complementaries of its neighbours. Contrast effect is greatest at the boundary of two colours; and it is the greater the more extended and saturated these are; it is also much more distinct when their contours have been masked by distance, by dispersion (in shadows), by the superposition of tissue paper, or by rotation in discs. Otherwise it is often hard for a person to detect the changes produced by contrast, especially when the contours of the colours are sharply defined. We seem to abstract from the super-induced change and to apprehend to some extent what the real colour of a surface is.

If we made a figure like the colour figure out of the four

sensations of the skin, putting one at each corner of a square and distant from its centre in proportion to its *intensity*, this centre would represent the lapse of all sensation. Each sensation would fade out as we approached this point. Let us suppose we were reducing warmth gradually. The intensity of the skin-sensation of the moment would not be kept up to a constant level in spite of this loss of warmth, say by the automatic proportional increase of its opposite cold. With the decrease of the " saturation " of warmth (or its loss of intensity) we should simply be the nearer to lapse of sensation altogether. Now let us imagine the same process for vision. As white gradually faded out, probably by an intensive change, its place would not be taken by black, thus making a darker and darker grey that would more or less steadily saturate the area in question with sensation. The white would rather gradually fade away, growing thinner and thinner until it was invisible. Then no visual sensation would be present at all. Proceeding beyond this central point of no colour, we should begin to see the thinnest trace of black, and so on to deepest black. The black from start to finish would be the same kind of black, just as the warmth would be. If colours really behaved thus in mixture, it would be easy to make a thing invisible, even if every material particle had to have some colour or other. We should only need to speckle it over with complementary spots. At a distance there would be no colour over all at all—on the present supposition.

But the mixture of complementaries actually leads only to a weakening of the dominant colour of the pair, until in the case of complete mutual annulment grey remains alone. Vision gives us no colour silence, as it were. The question then is: where does this perpetual day-long sensation come from? Not from the retina of the eye: for there the processes of red and green, of blue and yellow, of white and black mutually annul one another in proportion to their strength, and can just balance one another out altogether. The suggestion has been made that it is the brain that thus continually maintains visual sensation, generally grey of some degree: so that when our eyes are shut or when a part of the retina has been destroyed by inflammation, or in temporary or even permanent blindness, there is darkness, i.e. we see a black field of vision or a part of it. Light stimulation from the eye merely changes this central constant in its own direction; and the blackest black is not obtained by shutting off all light from the eye, but by means of contrast with a very bright background. The negative character of the black stimulus makes it impossible to get a black to be so intense as the white of direct sunlight. Very likely the action of this cerebral grey is the reason why differences of intensity are not apparent in the ordinary work of vision and why the field of vision is always full of colour, so that even the blind-spot does not make a gap in it.

It is commonly held that there are two systems of sense-organs in the retina—the cones and the rods. With the latter we see only the colours of the white-black series; the rods come into function only in light of low intensity: their threshold is some 1400–8000 times lower than that of the cones which serve the purpose of daylight vision. Nocturnal animals are abundantly supplied with rods for twilight vision, diurnal ones with cones. The fovea centralis contains only cones. Some totally colour-blind persons have only rod vision, their cones being apparently inactive. According to Edridge-Green, however, the rods are concerned solely with the formation and distribution of the visual-purple. This is the medium for stimulation of the cones which are the only receptors of vision. The visual-purple "trickles" into the fovea from the surrounding parts; without this supply it is blind. In dark adaptation the visual-purple accumulates and so vision becomes far more sensitive. Were the purple entirely used up, vision must completely lapse.

For the purposes of pure psychology the study of vision is at present rather ungratifying. An immense amount of the most patient investigation, both experimental and speculative, has been devoted to it. But there seems to be little or no hope of reaching a theory or explanation that is not purely physiological. Every analysis reduces the tri-dimensional continuum of colour qualities to a number of discreet primaries, each of which is correlated with some hypothetical process in the eye or the connected nervous system. None of the theories offers any prospect of understanding the nature of colour in itself. Photo-chemical theories [1] of colour suggest that a "mixed" colour like orange is really a field stippled irregularly all over with minute particles of pure red and pure yellow, corresponding to the photo-chemical atoms that at any moment are reacting in the "red" way or in the "yellow" way, whatever they are. But can we do anything psychologically to confirm them, except to agree that, for all we can tell, it may be so? Orange, then, would be like heat, if heat is nothing more than the simultaneous excitation of all the cold and warm spots of an area, as seems very probable. Only the granulation of the particles, so to speak, must be enormously finer. But it is just as true to say that orange merely resembles both red and yellow.

Perhaps in the facts of colour-contrast there is a faint glimmer of hope. The ordinary person finds it often quite difficult to see a contrast colour, and is quite surprised at the amount of it, when he has learned to see it. There seem to be two ways of looking at colour—the ordinary way and, let us say, the artistic way. The latter surely sees colour much more as the "eye" sees it. But in ordinary life we learn to modify our apprehension of colour to suit the circumstances. We seem to a surprising extent to abstract from the colour induced by contrast, from the colour of the atmosphere or other medium through which we see an object, from reflected light and the like. When we look at a snow-clad mountain that still holds the rays of the setting sun, we often see it as a white surface illuminated by red light, though sometimes this analysis fails and then the mountain seems to our great wonder to be clad in blood-red snow. Clouds always seem to have the colour of the light they reflect. To the ordinary man the colour judgments of the artist's pictures seem to be absurdly exaggerated or even perversely untruthful. These facts suggest that we are to some extent able psychically to move about within colour, so to speak, "seeing" or attending to one resemblance or component of it more

[1] These are now being displaced by theories of electronic resonance in conformity with recent work on atomic structure.

than to another, in the same general way in which we listen to one current of sounds (e.g. speech) rather than to accompanying noises. Other relevant and suggestive facts occur in connexion with binocular colour-mixture, especially when the areas of colour so presented only partially overlap and are severally well defined. The analysis of colour is greatly affected by the perception of these forms and by the perceptual recognition of the different surfaces or sources to which the components belong. So we can distinguish between the proper colour of a surface, the illuminating colour it reflects and the

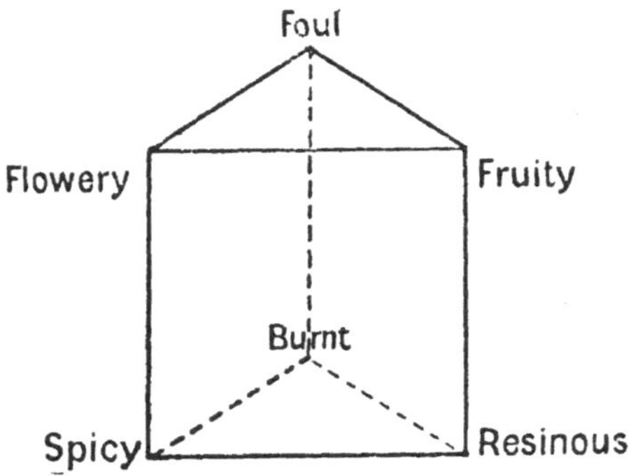

FIG. 5.

colour of the atmosphere it is seen through. The pleasure or displeasure evoked by juxtaposed colours also suggests that colours have some psychological, as well as merely physiological, kinship.

The psychological problem of colour-quality forms part of that of quality in general. And we need hardly expect to find a line of analytical progress more easily here than elsewhere. But we must keep on pressing till we succeed in penetrating the obscurity of quality.

The sense of smell offers quite as much material for our energies as vision. A diagrammatic survey of its qualities has recently been planned by Henning [1] in the form of a regular prism (Fig. 5). The odours that lie on the edge of the prism resemble only the two that occupy the end points of that edge, according to their distance from the latter. Examples of transitional smells are: spicy-

[1] *Ztsch. Psych.*, 1915–16, **73** to **76**.

flowery—thyme and vanilla, flowery-fruity—geranium, fruity-resinous—the piney odours, resinous-foul—fish scales, burnt-spicy—roasted coffee, foul-spicy—garlic, spicy-fruity—peppermint. Those that lie on a surface bear resemblance similarly to the four corners of that surface. There is no annulment or contrast as there is between colours. Mixture of smells always yields a true mixture of the qualities of the separate substances, not a quality intermediate between these as in the case of colour; mingled odours retain their individuality as in the case of simultaneous tones in a chord.

Differences of intensity are, of course, familiar in this sense, but there is little or no trace of any variation in either the position or the extent of smells. Some smells we call heavy, some light and ethereal: this may indicate some difference of mass or volume in smell. All smells seems to keep the same position relatively to one another.

This sense's chief work is to start the process of digestion; not, as has often been said, merely to warn us what is good and what not; but, if the food is good, to help us to recognise its presence and to excite the flow of saliva and of gastric juice, which are important agents of digestion.

In this work smell is closely allied with the chemical sense of taste, which is characterised by four distinctive qualities—sweet, sour, salty, bitter. The relations of these qualities are probably best expressed by a tetrahedron, having sweet, sour, and bitter at the corners of one side and salty at the fourth corner (H. Henning). When a sweet substance is mixed with a salty one the resulting taste seems not to be two qualities of sensation, but one that resembles both sweet and salt, as orange resembles red and yellow. And single substances may also give such tastes. Similarly for bitter-salt, sour-sweet, etc. Sensitivity to the four tastes is distributed over areas of the upper surface of the tongue that are not wholly coincident for any two. Taste thus bears resemblance both to vision and to the skin senses in their general psychophysical arrangements. Alkaline taste is really the smell of methylated ammonia (a product of the decomposed epithelium of the mouth).

CHAPTER VI

SENSATIONS IN GENERAL

WE may now make a Table (2) of the chief senses showing how the six attributes of sensation are varied in each of them. The senses have been arranged with regard to various useful groupings of them and to some of the resemblances of their qualities.

This table fulfils the purpose of the psychological study of elementary sensations as well as may be at present. It shows that sensation in general approximates to the type defined by the six attributes enumerated. It is probable that every sensation possesses some quality and can vary to some degree or other in intensity and in both systemic and temporal position as well as extent. Sometimes the evidence for this uniformity is vague and uncertain, as with the intensity of vision, the position of muscular sensations, and the systemic dimension of smell. But these are isolated breaks in our acquaintance with sense which may yet be filled in by careful experiment and observation. It is only in smell that we seem to find no trace of the missing attributes. And smells must surely have some position; for they are always located more or less vaguely about the nostrils: and location implies "position," although that can vary only very little for the different smells.

The special characteristics of the various senses seem to be explained by the following four sets of circumstances.

(1) *The amount of variation of each attribute.* This will in all probability depend upon the physical and physiological conditions of the sense. Thus the restriction of the regio olfactoria and the mode of access to it hardly leave physical room for variation of "position" or of extent in smell. The variations found in tone involve the existence of different stimuli as well as the special physiological apparatus of hearing.

(2) The number of minimal spots or particles of sensation that make up *the extent or size of area of the sensations*

TABLE 2. THE ATTRIBUTES OF SENSATION

The senses in various groupings			To what degree is each attribute variable					
					Systemic		Temporal	
			Quality	Intensity	Position	Extent	Position	Extent
General	Exteroceptive (outer)	Pain		Always	Very clearly		Not sharply	
		Warmth					,,	,,
		Cold	As a general rule				,,	,,
		Pressure	"One sense one quality"				Fairly sharp	
	Proprioceptive (inner)	Articular		Except here		(not here)	Very clearly	
		Muscular			Except here		Not clearly	
Special	Interoceptive (inner)	Hunger			,,	,,	,,	,,
		Thirst			,,	,,	,,	,,
		and others			,,	,,	,,	,,
	Exteroceptive (complex)	Sound					Very clearly	
		Sight	6 simple types	and here			Very clearly	
		Smell	6 simple types		and here		Not clearly	
		Taste	4 simple types		(Vaguely)		,,	,,

we commonly receive from each sense. Thus in warmth and cold and hunger these extents are usually very large,

5

in touch they are oftener nearly pointed, while in sounds there is always some characteristic size of area or volume.

(3) *The intensive grading of the particles* within the area. We have already referred to Bernstein's theory of intensive grading within the elementary spot of sensation and we have seen how grading in the large masses of sound and areal skin sensations distinguishes tone from noise and even from uneven. This grading over large extents implies the summation of intensities between, and it may be, over the centres of neighbouring spots, similar to that

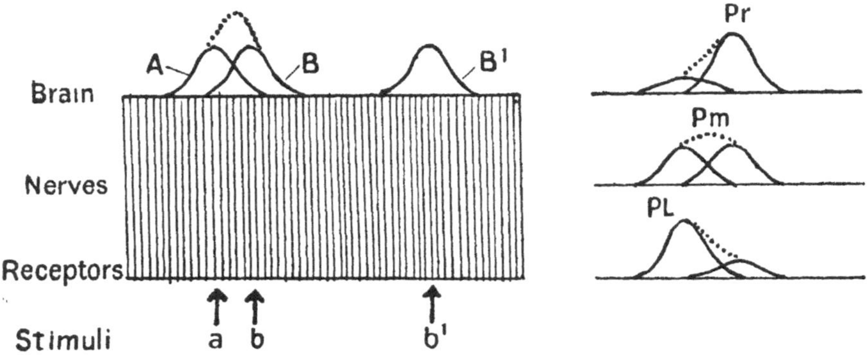

FIG. 6.—Each receptor is supposed to be linked to a certain spot of the cortex, as it must be *effectively*, although this linkage need not be exclusive *anatomically*.

which underlies the fusion of evenly distributed areal sensations.

An important case of Bernstein's theory for which it was, in fact, originally devised, is the production of a single spot of sensation (e.g. of touch) with only one inherent position, by the simultaneous stimulation of two receptors, standing it may be some considerable distance apart in the sensory field. It is represented in Figure 6, where *a* and *b* are the stimuli and A and B the sensations that would result from them, were they applied separately and successively. When *a* and *b* are as far apart as *a* and b^1 in the figure, the sensations they evoke would be quite distinct and two. When they are applied as *a* and *b* in the figure, their sensations would summate to form a single broader and centrally more intensive sensation; but only one position would predominate in it. Lesser extents of overlapping produced by separating the stimuli gradually would produce effects that may easily be verified in the sense of touch. Between a distinctly single, through larger and more intense, spot of touch and two separate spots we may observe a blunt point or circle, an oval or line of touch, and a dumb-bell form, in which two maxima are connected by sensation.

This simple scheme explains also why, on some parts of the skin, e.g. the shoulder, two points may be actually far apart and yet on successive stimulation may be "judged" the same.[1] It is a matter of indifference how far apart physically the contributory organs may lie, so long as there is centrally this overlapping or coincidence of excitations. And there is room for considerable practice in observation, just as in the case of the gradations between two clear points and one. It also explains why two sublimal stimuli, placed approximately, may produce a sensation[2]; and why the more intense of two stimulations seems to draw the less intense towards it.[3] But a more intense stimulation may absorb or inhibit a simultaneous weaker one. It also explains why the average error of localisation of points on the skin is less than the two point threshold and bears no direct relation to the latter.[4] And the accuracy of localisation of the different skin qualities follows the average density of their points, namely, pain (best), touch, cold, and warmth.[5] This accuracy is not improved by practice, though the two point threshold is. In this case repeated observation probably reveals two distinguishable maxima, which through carelessness or lack of practice were previously taken as one "lump."

In uniaural hearing a similar case is provided by simultaneous tones of neighbouring pitch. But it is complicated by the periodicity of the sound stimulus and by the formation of beats. Many tones of neighbouring pitch sounded

[1] Lufkin, op. cit.
[2] Brückner, *Ztsch. Psych.*, 1901, **26**, 33 ff.
[3] Cook and von Frey, *Ztsch. Biol.*, 1911, **56**, 537 ff.
[4] S. I. Franz, *Psych. Rev.*, 1913, **20**, 107 ff.
[5] M. Ponzo, *Arch. Ital. de Biol.*, 1913, **60**, 218 ff.

together give a sound of the pitch of the resultant average rate of vibration. When two tones of a larger interval, e.g. a third, fourth, etc., are sounded together, no new apex is formed, as the predominant points of the tones lie too far apart from one another. Each pitch can then be singled out by the attention in spite of the overlapping of the two masses. But it is obvious that the lower tone will more easily drown the higher one when this has been made weak than conversely.

(4) *The sharpness of definition* of the particles. The more sharply defined the sensation is, compared with the stimulus, the less scope will there be for fusion of points by overlapping and for displacement by relative changes of intensity. On the skin two points are more easily distinguished the more intense they are, so that the distance between them seems greater (Cook and von Frey, *ibid.*). Two distinct simultaneous points, on the contrary, attract one another, as it were, making the distance between them seem smaller than it seems on distinctly successive presentation. Possibly we then judge, not by the centre of the spot, as we should for a single spot, but by the distance between the nearer edges of the spots. We take the inner measure of them, so to speak. In senses like vision and touch greater sharpness of definition marks off a region of special sensitivity, the fovea and the finger tips. Vision, especially, then seems to be almost perfect; it practically reaches the limits set by the receptive surface of the retina. Contact of spots rather than overlapping is the rule here.

Clearness of definition, in relation to the cerebral process of sensation rather than to the number of elementary receptors, should be of great importance in the determination of the sensory powers of different animals. For as greater cerebral definition doubtless needs more room, we must expect to find the best discrimination of sensations where there is the biggest brain surface for any sense and generally where there is the biggest and most convoluted brain. An animal might have a very fine sense organ and all the nerve fibres for dealing with it centrally; but it would surely be incapable of the finest sensory work if these fibres were crowded or confused in a small area of brain surface. All sorts of variations must, of course, occur. The central parts of the nervous system are the prepared medium of all learning and training. In different species and individuals some sensory organs are more frequently used and call more urgently for discrimination. These should therefore usurp to themselves a fuller representation centrally. They might in time be brought much nearer to the physiological limit, as the sense of vision typically is in man. The experimental study of animal behaviour shows that the bigger the brain, the faster, more complex and general is the capacity for learning.

These four factors enable us to see how the senses can be so different in scope and delicacy, although they are all built upon the same general psychophysical plan. Our senses are no doubt primarily adapted to the world we live in. There may be various limitations to them inherent in the physiological constitution of the body itself, although they are not very apparent. Comparison of the senses of different animals shows us that the general mode of life and the typical needs of each species call for modification of the senses. To some extent, however, the converse may be the primary agent : the structure of the senses may determine the mode of life. The question is intrinsically subtle and complex. If we had been bred in a very different environment from this world, our senses would doubtless have been very different too. Temperature and smell might have been the " higher " and " far " senses while sight and sound might have been very lowly forms, as they are actually in the worms and insects respectively. If we had an area of the most delicate touch, say about a foot square in size, we could create for it an art of form that would take rank beside the best of our arts.

We are now able to set out the notion of psychophysical parallelism in the form in which it can be established with the greatest precision. This notion implies that the physical and psychical elements or processes—here of sensation and by hypothesis of experience in general—correspond point for point. Every elementary receptor that can be separately stimulated evokes from the (normal) nervous system its own little particle of sensation. The excitation from each receptor is carried forward into the central nervous system in a complicated way. But we have no reason to suppose that it is there scattered and dissipated until it has done the work necessary for the occurrence of sensation. A change of position in the sensation corresponds to a change of locus in the receptor-neural process. A change in the number of (neighbouring) sensory particles corresponds to a change in the number of (neighbouring) receptor-neural processes. An increase of sensory intensity follows an increase of neural intensity. If there be some doubt—on the basis of the physiological rule of "all or nothing" for neurones, whether this is always true in relation to the receptor, it will, nevertheless, hold for the central process. Processes of summation of unitary contributions must there provide a basis for differences of intensity in sensation.

From these explicit grounds for the notion of psychophysical parallelism we may go on to postulate that a change of sensory quality indicates a change in some other aspect of the central process. And similarly for the temporal attributes. But we have not yet the slightest idea what these aspects are. Much has still to be done before the theory of psychophysical parallelism is completed. But it would be pedantically sceptical to refuse to acknowledge its great probability as a general plan of the senses.

Quality is the attribute that gives us the least hope of insight into itself. Some qualities resemble one another more than others, e.g. those of vision (or of taste) than those of pain, touch, and warmth. But we have no sort of clue to the system in which all the qualities known to us stand, nor have we any sort of psychological theory of any set of qualities of any sense, be it vision or smell, taste or temperature. The most that can be done is to arrange the qualities according to resemblance to one another, as our various diagrams have shown. But we are quite unable to step beyond this descriptive knowledge to any truly psychological analysis of quality. Probably each distinctive quality of sensation represents a single (physiological) sense. This is always clearly stated for the outer and inner senses and it is implied in the construction of most colour theories. In the sense of smell it has not yet been carried through with any semblance of success, though it was attempted by Zwaardemaker. The systemic attributes seem far more intelligible to us, doubtless because they suggest this idea of parallelism and confirm it the more we pursue it into its details. And quality seems so mysterious because it offers no sign whatever of any parallelism. It looks, on the contrary, like something quite new, something that matter could hardly produce by itself: for, as far as we know, all differences of matter are reducible to differences of spatial arrangement and movement of particles of one or more unknown kinds. Intensity is not quite so strange, in spite of its (psychical) indivisibility and immeasurability. For it feels like quantity; and the physical concept of intensity involves either number-density or speed. The temporal attributes, finally, also seem understandable, because we think we measure time physically.

Strictly speaking (or philosophically), we must recognise that none of the attributes is any worse or better than any other. Time only exists mentally, as an individual "thing": physically it is an unknown quantity that separates, or rather, is implicit in events (as they are reconstructed in independence of any particular point of observation, by the theory of relativity). The same is true of space. So the mystery of quality seems less oppressive. Nevertheless, it is (unphilosophically) true to say that quality is more mysterious than the others, as it suggests the presence in nature of a kind of unknown that is not detectable by any physical means.

Working forward from the idea of a parallelism between the elements of sense and receptor-neural processes, we may proceed to the assumption that *all* experience is bound by some such neural general plan to its neural basis in the cerebral cortex. This seems already a more probable theory of the connexion between mind and body than does animism or interactionism, the action of the brain upon the mind or soul as a whole. Here a psychic being or soul is postulated: and the total sensory "content" of consciousness at any moment represents the complex response of the soul to many simultaneous cerebral influences, which may be qualitatively distinct and spatially separate processes. The soul responds in its own unique, and always unitary, way. It is true indeed that mind and matter seem to be entirely different kinds of things. But when we recognise this, we usually forget that we have not the least idea what sort of a thing (or " essence ") matter is, whereas we can directly observe the essence of consciousness in general and of its different types in particular (e.g. blue, extent, solid, concept, certainty, etc.). Of matter we know only a great deal about the forms, arrangements, and movements of its units. And we are by no means unable to distinguish *different* units of complication amongst our experiences. We are not limited solely to the unity of the mind (or soul) as a whole, though that is a very important problem, of course. Hence whatever we may yet have to learn about these unities, we have already established a highly probable correspondence between simplest facts of mind and facts of body : namely, between differences of sensation and such physical differences of receptor and nerve as we can distinguish. We should make this knowledge our base-line for the further exploration of psychophysical relations. If we keep true to the proportions of things, there can be no fear of our letting mind degenerate into a mere reflexion of matter or mechanism. For we know much more qualitatively about mind than about matter. And one of these important facts is that mind is essentially coherent and only secondarily, if at all, mechanical, as matter seems to us entirely to be (probably because we cannot see the coherence or spirit of it).

Thus we see how important it is to study the system inherent in experience, i.e. to distinguish its differences in all their detail, as we have done with the elements of sensation ; to bring these differences into connexion with one another, as we have done by comparing the different senses with one another ; and thereby to win, as it were, the secret of the constitution of mind. In time we may be able to say whether we have already run through the whole gamut of its possibilities, or whether fields of mind may lie beyond our present horizon. This is one of the problems that makes pure psychology so fascinating a study and that lends it some of the charms of the macrocosm of astronomy and the microcosm of physics. The study of the mind in action is of great value for the needs of practice. But it can never be really successful until we know exactly what the mind is that is involved in action. That is just what we have already shown—that the successful study of psychophysics implies some co-ordinate success, both in the study of (pure) psychology and in the study of physiology. There is no short cut to psychophysics over or under these two.

CHAPTER VII

THE GENERAL TYPES OF INTEGRATION. SYSTEMIC DISTANCE

HAVING brought the elements of sense into their most probable order, which proves on the whole to be tolerably simple, we must turn our attention to experiences that are characteristic of the unified grouping or integration of these elements. We naturally expect these integrations to show an orderly connexion with the system of elements and themselves to form an orderly system. Our problem is like that of a chemist who discovers something about the elements that compose material substances; he will not fail to wonder whether these elements obey similar laws in the compounds they form. Or like the biologist we may enquire whether the elements of sense *evolve* in any way into the higher states of mind with which our practical interests are commonly engaged. We all know so much about evolution, if only in a popular way, that we expect the progress of evolution to be orderly and not erratic.

In many ways these expectations are fulfilled. We find good reason to believe that mind, like nature, is built on a coherent plan and works in an orderly way. Or being founded upon, or consisting of, certain elements, the integrations it shows flow from the nature and properties of these elements and are therefore as systematic as the latter. The plans of mind are not those of the material system, to be sure. Nor can its actions be said to be merely mechanical. But they seem to share in that systematic coherence and rationality that in nature so gratifies our love of knowledge.

The attributes of quality and intensity show hardly any sign of evolution or of integration. This seems rather to be the special virtue of the attributes of position, both systemic and temporal. And of these two the systemic attributes, especially position, integrate very much farther than the temporal. We may, in fact, hazard the guess that the whole system of cognitive experience, ending in connected thought or trains of reasoning, is the product of the integration of these attributes. It is built upon, and consists of, the successive syntheses of these attributes. And in the end it resembles a complication of the attribute of systemic position more than anything else.

The simpler integrations of systemic position are known as systemic form. When two pressure-contacts are set some distance apart on the skin (cf. *a* and b^1 in Fig. 6) we notice the presence not only of the two spots of sensation, but of another sensory datum, namely, the *distance* between them. We are prone to think that we somehow merely estimate or reckon by thought the distance between such points. But that must be a mistaken view. There seems to be no means by which reason could make two spots of sensation produce a distance between them. Nor could we by any logic educe this distance from the attributes of these spots. We seem forced to admit distance as new datum, adding something uniquely new to all that appertains to the two spots. But at the same time it is perfectly clear that the spots and the distance are bound together into a special whole, so that we must speak of the spots and their distance or of the distance between the spots. This special synthesis we shall call integration, and it is important to notice carefully what is involved in the notion, namely, (1) something new that is the essence or "spirit" of the unity, and (2) the peculiar unity of the whole whereby the integrating parts and the new thing (or "integrate") are wrought indissolubly together, and are attached or refer to one another. It is tempting at once to ponder over the nature of the bond between the integrants and the integrate. But it would be rash to do so before we have won some idea of the system of integrations of which this seems to be the first. From consideration of the whole, when we approximately attain to it, we shall probably gain greater insight into each than from the most intensive study of any one.

We are able to compare distances readily with one another in almost complete independence of the particular identity of the spots upon which they are founded. Size is the comparable characteristic of distances. Distances, like intensities, constitute a series of magnitudes which cannot be strictly and essentially measured. They can only be arranged in order of magnitude. But it is easy to place between any two spots another so that the distances from the latter to either of the former shall be equal. Nevertheless, even when the middle spot is made to lie on the line joining the others, this operation does not strictly divide the unitary distance between the outside spots into two, so that we may say the former is psychologically twice as great as the latter. For the unity of any distance is strictly indivisible. And we should still have to ascertain by experiment whether the larger distance, were it psychologically divisible, would necessarily appear to be exactly twice the distance produced by this physical or mathematical division. But we can truly say that the divided distance is half the undivided distance, if we remember that this division implies the creation of two smaller distances by the insertion of another spot, and the judgment of their equality. "Double" in this (real) sense has a very precise meaning and value. In respect of the mere (phenomenal) arrangement of sizes in order of magnitude it has little value or precision.

The unity of distance is shown very clearly in the fact that the comparison of distances follows Weber's law, which we encountered in discussing the immeasurable magnitudes of intensity. If a standard distance is compared with a variable one by regular methods it is found that the line just noticeably greater than the standard physically exceeds the latter by a constant ratio. In comparing lines or distances for this purpose we must carefully avoid all the ordinary methods of measuring lengths. We must not place the lines against one another so that we can subtract one from the other or the like. They must be kept apart, so that we see each clearly as a whole.

In certain senses, especially in touch and vision, the constant practice of everyday life has made our discrimination keen and our analysis psychologically true and sufficient. In these senses the systemic field is of simple construction and the sensations are often clearly divided into distinct patches. In them, therefore, we readily learn the connexion between distance and spots of sensation of different position. Notions thus won from the simpler senses may, as in our study of the elements of sense, stand as a hypothesis by which we may test and control our analysis of the other senses. And we therefore expect to find some sort of distance in every sense in which differences of systemic position occur freely along with some definition of the separate points. Conversely, if we find in these other senses differences that show kinship with the distances of touch and vision, then the attribute which must vary in the sensations required for these distances will have to be classed as systemic and positional. By this method we are led to recognise several chief senses of form, namely, vision and articular sense, in lesser degree touch, and in a special manner hearing.

In the articular sense distances are given in the finest detail and they must bear the same relation to the positions inherent in the elementary sensations as is so plainly evident in vision. This confirms our previous conclusion that the chief variant of articular sense is the attribute of position and not that of quality. Articular sensation also draws our attention to a further general feature of integration, namely, that the sensations constituting the integration need not always be simultaneous (as visual forms so typically are). They may appear *in succession*, provided the interval between them is not too long. In articular sense successive presentation is the rule for any one joint. A joint can occupy only one physical position, and so can give only one sensory position, at a time.[1] Only as between different joints, e.g. those of the fingers, do we get a complex of simultaneous distances.[2] And if we use the fingers of both hands along with other joints and limbs, distances in three different dimensions are quite clearly present

[1] We shall discuss the question of motion, which seems to involve more than one position at a time, later on.

[2] A very striking presentation of distance is given in Aristotle's familiar illusion and in other similar displacements of parts of the skin surface.

simultaneously. A single joint hardly gets beyond the single dimension it occupies, unless we think of the circular motions of which the ball-and-socket joints are capable. The great form-capacity of the articular sense puts it alongside the visual sense as the other most important sensory constituent of the human mind. Vision, however, attains the greater mastery over three dimensions. And these two senses working conjointly in further integrations seem to provide the essential basis upon which the pinnacle of mind in thought and reason ultimately rises.

In the sense of sound the attribute of position appears in the pitch of tones, as we have seen. Different pitches are therefore a certain distance apart. But we have little power of comparing these distances, for, as we shall see, the proportions between the volumes of tones are so much more important than the distances between their pitches that we pay all attention to the former and none to the latter. Besides, as all tones are built of sound-particles beginning from the " high " end of the series and proceeding downwards as far as need be to constitute their volume, the higher must always overlap the lower. So although the pitches mark out certain points or partials, these are always surrounded by sensation. Thus the feature of pure distance, which stands out alone, as it were, between distant points of touch or vision, is here rather lost in lengths or areas of sensation.

In this pure state distance is like the ideal straight line—length without breadth. But there is also the actual straight line. This may be considered as an outgrowth of the extent of the sensory spot or as many minimal spots in a continuous series. Distance is, of course, latent in the single spot of sensation, although it is not evident in its pure form until it rests upon such minimal extents of very different " position."

If the actual straight line is extended in the other dimension, we have area of sensation, which is also latent in the single " spot." In an area there are an infinite number of distances, of course. But that need cause us no more psychological difficulty than did the infinity of positions that is ideally present in a spot of sensation or in a " motion." We can look upon the great variety of distances as latent in an area and as made patent when we draw a real or imaginary line through the area or mark out one special distance by some such means, e.g. by special spots at two places in the area. In this way distance or the ideal straight line may be looked upon as the absolutely final element of all integrations of form or figure, no matter how complex they are. Of course as a special phase of experience distance is best reserved for the name of the "essence" that unifies two very different sensory spots; whereas extent is the name of the kindred aspect of continuous sensation from one spot to another. But, of course, the two terms meet ultimately in the idea of real infinitely divisible particles of sensation having the properties named by the attributes. As we have seen we need to carry on our psychological notions mathematically in this way, just as physicists carry on theirs, always under the due constraint of the facts of their science.

It is evident (cf. p. 25) that the whole nature of every figure is fully determined by the elementary sensations of which it consists along with the distances that emerge from their more or less distant positions. This is the total *conformation* of the figure, in which all the component elements are preserved without loss. We do not need, therefore, to attribute to the figure any further integrative aspect to constitute its figure or conformation. Even if considerable psychological work must be done if we are to distinguish one figure from the wider conformation in which it stands and to adjust ourselves actively in some way to it, this implies only a process in some other region or level of mind or mind-body relations, for which the basis is in this level of sensory complication already fully supplied. We need see no peculiar act of figure-forming or of step-forming or of comparison or of "step" (simply) in the sensory stuff. The notions of (1) elementary sensations, (2) attributes, (3) fusion, and (4) the resulting conformation by summative overlapping are all that we need. There is no reason why elementary sensations should be supposed to be in themselves indivisible and mutually repellent, if the facts of sensation indicate the contrary. These elements are for us merely the *natural* "spots" or units in which extent is only faintly evident and distances not at all. The mutual interaction of neighbouring areas (cf. p. 17), on the other hand, is merely an incident of their contact or fusion. That interaction is therefore present in the conformation before any attention or comparison of parts can be undertaken. And there seems to be no reason why an animal, fowl, chimpanzee, child or man, should not adjust its actions to several aspects or parts of a conformation at once, as well as to one small areal sensation or to an elementary particle. For in learning to respond to the intenser or brighter or larger of two areas, its responses to the one are favoured and to the other disfavoured. When the smaller magnitude is then replaced by a still larger one, it shows this " set " of action by responding usually positively to the latter, not to the former (larger) as an individual, absolute, clue. It takes longer to " forget " the disfavoured one than we had supposed. But how long, or under what conditions, we do not yet know. And after all the double " yes-no " attitude, to which the conformation corresponds, must be very present to the learner in the early stages of his successful adjustment.

Whether it be due to the nature of distance as the ideal straight line of experience or not, we have a very fine sense for any deviation from the true straight line of continuous (visual) sensation. In this respect vision displays its usual expertness. The lengths of markedly curved lines are very hard to estimate and to compare. Degree of curvature is reckoned by observation of the angle formed with the curve by an imaginary straight line joining its ends. We are so skilled in constructing these lines that we often seem actually to see the lines we imagine. Our sense for straightness in articular sense, especially in the joints of the arms, is also notable.

The senses seem to be specially organised so as to heighten the outline of areas of sensation. Visual artists are fond of asserting that visual " masses " have no outline. But though there may be no such thing *ultimately* as mathematical or physical (or, in accordance with the suggestions of the previous paragraph but one, even psychological) outline, there certainly is outline in the ordinary psychological sense of the term. In fact, it is an aspect of areal sensations that is often as distinct, and as easily apprehended as any other, if not more so. Visual outlines are heightened by colour contrast, while in touch the parts most clearly marked out in a mass are those where there is a rapid change of pressure over a small area, i.e. again the outlines. The inner parts disappear by physical and neural adaptation. When the arm is plunged into water and moved up and down in it, we feel the pressure most distinctly at its surface like a ring of touch around the arm. For various purposes of art, however, it is doubtless more important to lay stress upon mass and its quality (colour) than upon outline. No phenomenon of outline has been established for articular sense or for hearing. In these senses sensations decrease gradually towards their borders.

This function of outline is probably closely connected with another general characteristic of figures, especially of visual figures. That is the relation of figure to the ground it stands upon. This has often been described as a function of attention: the figure is said to be at the focus of attention. This description seems to attribute a special "field" to attention, the relation of which to the fields of the several senses it would be difficult to describe. It seems far simpler to describe these functions as properties of the sensory complexes themselves. For even though they are undoubtedly affected by the work of attention (whether merely motor or "instinctive," or even conceptual), they are similar to the almost mechanical function of outline. This suggests that their basis is sensory and psychophysical and that it is merely altered (increased or decreased) by the process of attention.

Thus the four pairs of parallel lines along with the spaces between them (Fig. 7) form a "figure." But the white of the paper forms the ground on which they stand, and that white ground is continuous from the left beyond a to the right beyond d_1. The spaces between a and a_1, b and b_1, etc., form a more intimate vivid part of the

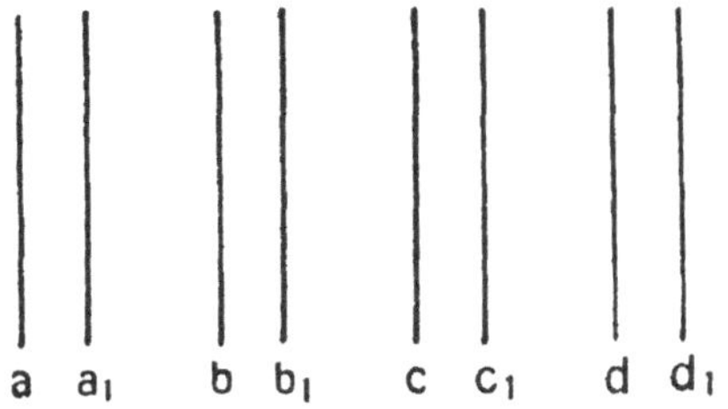

FIG. 7.

figure than the spaces between a_1 and b, b_1 and c.[1] These are merely the spaces between the different pairs aa_1, bb_1. This is more evident in the figure (Fig. 7a), where the spaces between the lines are all equal. We can apprehend these as four pairs of lines, but we can also readily see them as three pairs of lines and two single lines, or as two threes and two, or as two fours, or the like. As such groupings are made, so the spaces within the group seem to bind themselves into one with the lines bounding them and to leave hold of the nearest line of neighbouring groups. It is not nearly so easy to make the lines a_1b, b_1c, c_1d, of Fig. **7** form pairs as when the variously pairing lines are equally far apart.

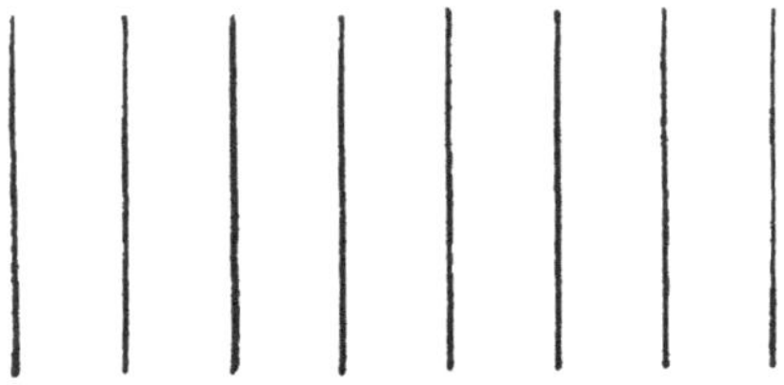

FIG. 7a.

There is, therefore, a greater liveliness in the figure than in the spaces between the figures or in the general background. These latter spaces seem relatively dead. They do not, of course, lose their character as distances : as such they remain as determinate as ever. But they are no longer components of a whole that stands out before us and engages the mind to further work, not only constituting itself by the inherent force of its own parts, but producing effects that reach farther forth into the mind's structure. The other spaces are components of this active whole and so seem more lively, more present and real, as it were. What these remoter effects are that constitute figure in this special sense, we shall consider later (p. 194 ff.).

So much life does such figure have, in fact, that it seems able to define forms that are as sensory areas partly indeterminate. This is familiar in silhouette advertisements where part of the figure is lost against a background like itself : and yet the " eye " induces an illusory line, carrying on the contour through the obscurity (cf. Fig. 8 [2]). Many " illusions " illustrate the interchangeability of

[1] Cf. K. Koffka, *Psych. Bull.*, 1922, **19**, 553 f.

[2] D. Starch, *Experiments in Educ. Psychology*, p. 151. New York, 1919.

figure and ground, especially those of reversible perspective (cf. Fig. 9). The shock of surprise with which we often discover the figure sought for in a " puzzle picture " shows how distinctive a thing for the observing mind a figure

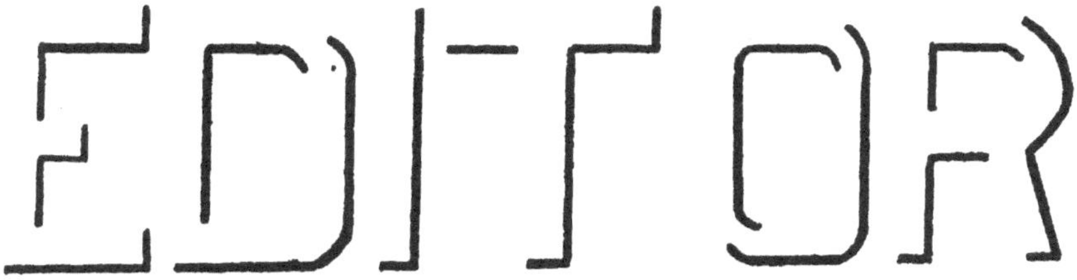

FIG. 8.

may be. It is hard to discover it, but once we have found it, we cannot " unsee " it again. And we can attend to the ground of such alternating figures, although the ground then readily assumes the characters of a figure, especially if our figure-habits predispose it to do so. At first the 6-7 cube figure may be seen for a long time in the one aspect, but after a few reversals it reverses very much more readily (Fig. 9). And it is quite difficult to *see* the cube figure as a set of intersecting lines on the surface of the paper. We know it is this really, but it is difficult to see it so flat as this.

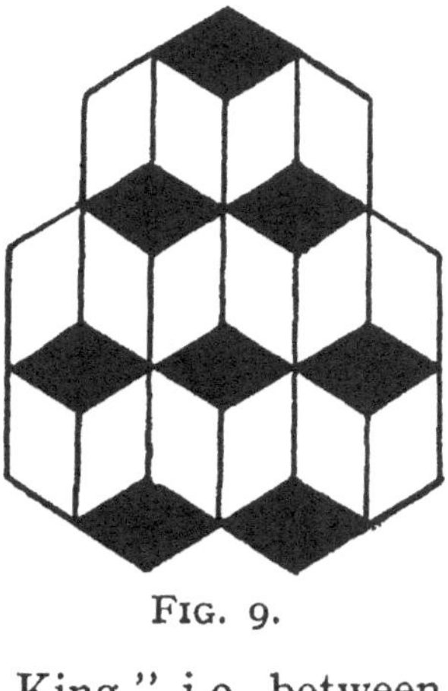

FIG. 9.

We find similar relations of figure and ground in the study of time-intervals and melody. The intervals of time between the first tones ra-ta-ta-tá of Mendelssohn's Funeral March form integral parts of this rhythmic figure: the time between this and its repetition is a mere lapse of time by comparison. It is the ground of time on which the music is played rather than a time-part of the music itself. Similarly the tones at the end of the third and the beginning of the fourth line of " God save the King," i.e. between " King " and " Send " rather constitute a mere change of pitch than an interval, a dead not a real interval, although as far as sensation goes they form an interval as well as the other tones do.

Other similar relations of ground and figure are found between the colour of an object and its surface-colour or the colour-atmosphere it stands in. They are particularly prominent in the processes of motion, as we shall see.

Although all parts of any visual figure are merely relative to one another, so that we might think it a matter of indifference how the figure is placed, yet we find that the inversion of a figure often makes it unrecognisable. And in spite of our familiarity with the visual form of copper-plate writing, it is by no means easy to write it backwards. In writing, a series of articular movements is made from left to right: if the left hand can make exactly the same series from right to left, the result is the mirror image of the former. But what a caricature the left hand's efforts seem when they are held up to view in front of a mirror! And yet there are exceptional persons to whom this mirror-writing comes easily and perfectly as a sudden discovery (after they have learnt to write with the right hand, of course). The others find it much easier to write with the left hand if they write at the same time with the right hand, i.e. if the movements are made symmetrically from the centre ("ambidextrously"). A scheme of control is thus provided, showing that it is rather the fixity of the visual standpoint to figure that accounts for the difficulty of writing than any special standpoint inherent in articular sense. Mirror-drawing, similarly, moving a pencil along the lines of a figure seen in a mirror and not directly visible, is also very difficult at first. But it is quite easy if the figure is held nearly flat on the top of the head while it is being traced out. The important, innately variable, difference of special dexterity of one hand points, however, to a general standpoint inherent in articular sense. It is impossible as yet to describe it simply or to trace it to a definite psychophysical source. But the left hand is very often used as a basis or ground for the more rapid and figure-like work of the right hand. The standpoint of vision seems to be determined by our constant interest in balance and stability and thereby in the vertical direction. But the peculiar variations of standpoint shown in the sense of touch by the act of writing letters on different parts of the skin with the blunt end of a pen or the like, show that these standpoints are many and various, depending greatly upon our physical orientation to the objects in question. But of their general presence there can be no doubt.

The existence of a special standpoint in hearing is shown by the difference between ascending and descending intervals. Those who have just learnt the former and easier, may be unable even then to recognise the same in descending order. Our standpoint towards tones may be described as central. The important point of tone is its centre or pitch and the centre of a mass of tones is the pitch of its lowest component. So the lowest partial of an instrumental blend gives the whole tone its nominal pitch. The bass voice is the most sonorous and influential of all in music. We naturally reckon intervals upwards from the lower tone, not downwards. Tones form (musically) a unidimensional field. Sounds in general resemble the lines of vision more than any other typical form.

The existence of general and special standpoints towards sensations does not require us to attribute corresponding " aspects " or " steps " or other structures to sensations. As already noted, a basis for such standpoints is sufficiently provided in the *conformation* of an extensive sensation and in the responses we establish for it. The conformation itself is not something new over and above the psychophysical aggregation that constitutes it.

CHAPTER VIII

PROPORTION

ONE of the most important relations between forms is their proportion. Without it we should be unable to recognise the identity of a figure that changes size under the influence of distance from the eye, or the like. Our sense of visual proportion seems to be very fine indeed ; it is even finer than our sense of difference between two lengths of line (Bühler). Our power to write in small or large letters even without the control of vision shows that proportion is strong in articular sense also.

In hearing proportion constitutes our sense of " interval." An interval, e.g. a major third, is one and the same proportion of tonal volumes. Since the volumes of tones decrease progressively from the lowest to the highest, it is evident that to any one volume another can always be found that bears to it the proportion given by any two volumes. A given interval, in other words, can always be repeated in any other part of the musical range of tone.

This theory of interval is based upon the following considerations—the first being certain familiar experimental facts regarding the fusion of tones. Pairs of instrumental or pure tones are played together, with special precautions against any indirect signs that two have been played rather than one (e.g. the noise of striking the notes, or noticeable succession, etc.). The subject, usually rather unmusical of course, is required to say whether he hears one, two, or more tones. It is found that the octave-pair very often passes for a single tone, the fifth less often, then in gradually decreasing amounts the fourth, the thirds and sixths, the tritone, minor seventh and major second, and the major seventh and minor second. The amounts are respectively 80, 50, 35 per cent for the octave, fifth, fourth, and thereafter from 30 per cent downwards in slowly decreasing amounts. Musical subjects, of course, often, if not always, hear and distinguish the tones that are present in each interval. And, if they are very expert, they can even name them at once without mistake. But these persons confirm the impression of apparent unity indicated in the answers of the unmusical by recognising in the octave the highest degree of apparent unity in the stuff of the tones as it were; in the fifth the next degree; in the fourth the third degree, and so on. Statistics got by comparing each interval with every other and saying which is the better fusion yield on the average the series: 8, 5, 4. III, 3, VI, 6, II, 7, 2, VII, where the Roman numbers mean the major intervals and the Arabic ones the minor ones and the consonances.

These facts of fusion are of decisive importance, because by holding for pure tones they show that the grades of musical consonance and dissonance are not brought about by any relations between the upper partials of the tones of an interval, as Helmholtz's theory of consonance proposed. It is true that, if every tone possessed the whole ideal series of harmonic partials, a tone an octave higher than another would have as its partials every second partial of the other tone, a tone a fifth higher would have every third partial of the other, a fourth higher would have every fourth partial, and so on. But it is precisely the tones that are most concerned with consonance and dissonance that do not possess the whole series of partials, all told. Instrumental tones, as we have seen, differ from one another in the selection from the ideal series of partials that they incorporate. If Helmholtz's theory were true, the same interval ought to differ in consonance from one musical instrument to another: which is absurd. His theory, moreover, begs the question: for it tacitly assumes that partials fuse with their fundamental to form an impression of one tone, which is the very phenomenon to be explained. And it holds only for successive tones, not for simultaneous ones. It is therefore untenable.[1]

[1] For a full discussion of Helmholtz's theory, see *The Foundations of Music*, 1920, Chapter VI.

By themselves grades of fusion are not explicable in any obvious way. But if they are set into relation to the general structure of tones and to their connexion with one another, an explanation arises that seems satisfactory. Every pure tone is a finely graded volume of sound with a single series of sound-particles, beginning always at the same " high " end of the series and extending downwards as far as need be to form the size of volume required. Hence the volume of any tone is always partially overlaid by the volume of any higher tone, as we have seen. Therefore when tones are sounded together, the following arrangement of volumes (among others) must occur (Fig. 10).

This constitutes the nearest possible approximation to the form of a single tone. For in the combined resultant

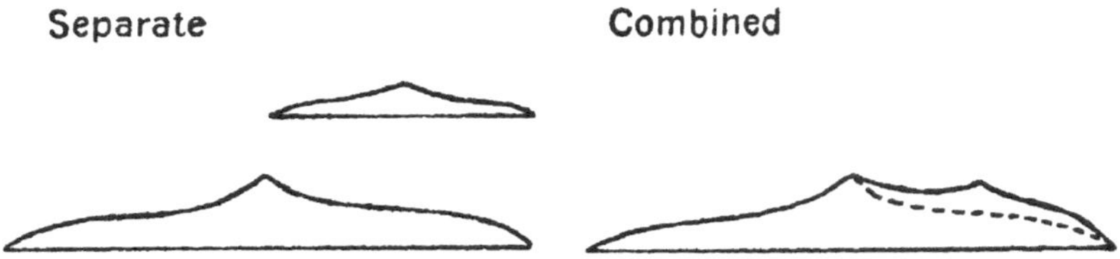

FIG. 10.

there is only one point at which the smooth grading of the pure or single tone is markedly disturbed, namely at the pitch of the higher tone. If we ascribe this arrangement to the octave, then the relations for the fifth, expressed in lengths of volumes, will probably be three for the lower and two for the higher tone. The overlapping of the tones now makes two points of departure from the intensive grading of a single tone, at equal distances from the pitch of the lower tone, namely, the pitch of the higher tone and the lower end of its volume. This produces a second degree of balance between tones and so a second approximation to the balance and symmetry of a single tone. Or the argument may be reversed: the overlapping of volumes by two parts upon three must some time occur, and it is evident that it contains an aspect of balance or of approximation to the unity and balance of a single tone; but the fifth is the fusion that next most resembles one tone; therefore in the fifth the overlapping of tones is two upon three parts, which is consistent with the octave being one upon two.

The relations which follow for the other intervals are such as yield characteristics appropriate to their musical functions. Thus in close dissonances, such as the minor and major second, the pitches of the two tones lie so close together that like two skin points they can be distinguished only with some difficulty. Between this range of dissonance due to *loss of distinction in confusion*, and the consonances (octave, fifth and fourth) which create a *loss of distinction in unity* we find a range in which the pitches of the two tones can be distinguished from one another with great ease. This range contains the musical intervals of the thirds and sixths. The other dissonances (the tritone, the sevenths, and the minor sixth in so far as it is dissonant or in its augmented-fifth form) are to be explained by their proximity to the great consonances (octave and fifth) and by the obvious lack of balance they show as compared with these. Their pitches are more readily distinguishable from one another than are those of the close dissonances. When the lower tone contains its first partial, as it very often does, it and the higher tone of a seventh or a ninth will show the same confusion as is seen in the close dissonances.

The infinite variety of intervals from unison to octave thus falls into various ranges whose characteristics are exemplified in the intervals music has chosen for its use. But the number of intervals rejected by music is much greater than is the number adopted. The latter must be favoured by special circumstances. Apart from the need for systematic coherence, which may be illustrated by the fact that major triads on C (c, e, g) on G (g, b, d) and on C downwards (f, a, c) mark out the whole diatonic scale, various other circumstances are influential in guiding selection.

First there are the difference-tones that accompany the interval and their distinguishability from one another and from the primary tones. The interval of a fifth produces a difference-tone an octave below the lower tone. This low tone fuses as octave with the lower tone of the interval and as (octave plus) fifth with the higher tone.

In the major third the difference-tones lie (a) two octaves and (b) a fourth, below the lower tone. In the minor third they lie (a) two octaves plus a major third and (b) a major third below the lower tone. The fusions of the major third are thus better than those of the minor, for thirds, as just noted, make more easily distinguishable tones than octaves and fourths. Thus the influence exerted by difference-tones is referable, apart from their mere number, to the relations of confusion and distinction that characterise pure tones. The same holds true in every respect for the upper partials that accompany the tones of an interval. They may coincide, and the more they do so, the greater is the unity produced. If they differ between the tones, they will introduce balance or confusion according to the intervals they form with one another and with primary tones. Of course they are usually themselves indistinguishable, so that they can only smoothen or roughen their tones. Lastly when tones are nearly of the same pitch, be they primary, partial, or differential tones, they form beats with one another ; as many beats per second, namely, as is the difference in the numbers of vibrations per second that correspond to their nominal pitches. Beats are essentially a fluctuation in the intensity of tone. Occurring in rapid succession they constitute another kind of confusion or roughness between tones. When difference-tones or partials fall into such pitches as give minimal amounts of beating, they make an interval that is *ceteris paribus* not only pleasanter to hear, but also more useful in connected music because it is easier for the ear to seize the pitches or tones it includes.

Figure 11 [1] shows the louder difference-tones for the range of an octave and a fifth. The ratio of vibrations for the tones of the diatonic scale are: 24, 27, 30, 32, 36, 40, 45, 48. The difference-tones for any combination of these tones can be easily calculated. They can readily be detected with a series of forks corresponding to the series of partials of a fundamental. The relative rates of vibration of these forks are, of course: 1, 2, 3, 4, 5, 6, 7, 8, 9, 10, etc. Any two neighbouring forks played loudly, will give (a) a loud tone h–l, of ratio 1, i.e. the lowest fork of

[1] C. Stumpf, *Ztsch. Psych.*, 1910, **55**, 1 ff.

the series: (b) played gently, a tone 2l–h, whose ratio in the series will be the next lower than the lower primary tone; (c) a tone 2h–l, the tone next above in the series; and (d) a tone h+l. For the interval of a major third (4 : 5) these difference-tones are respectively: (a) 1, (b) 3, (c) 6, (d) 9. If the ear is unable to find them, they may readily be proved to exist by making them beat with the tone of the corresponding fork slightly mistuned with a sliding weight.

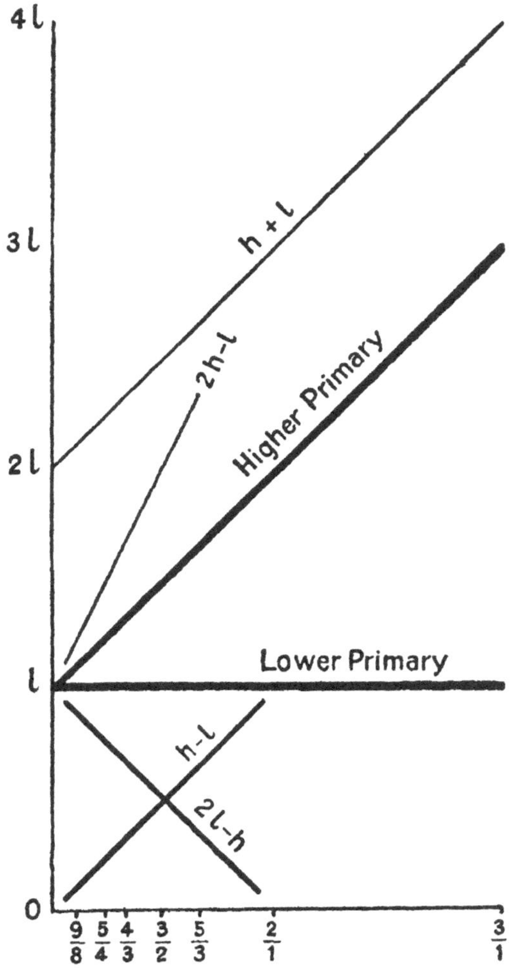

FIG. 11.—The thickness of the lines for each tone corresponds with its relative loudness. After Stumpf.

A given interval can be repeated with great ease throughout a considerable range of pitch, the most of which is represented on a good modern pianoforte. Here, as we have seen, the volumes of the tones of an interval are inversely proportional to the rates of physical vibration that evoke them. But at the upper end of this range the volumes remain increasingly too large for the rate of vibration, at the lower end too small, so that these high tones seem flatter and the low tones sharper than they should be. After being too flat at the higher limit by about a tone, judgment finally breaks down and the observer cannot indicate the pitch of a tone by absolute judgment (naming its pitch) or by transposition to a lower octave, even approximately. The reason for this is probably that the cochlea cannot take up tones of more than a certain wave-length, nor can the sensitive membrane respond with proper delicacy to impressions of less than a certain size. Thus we see that the range of musical hearing is naturally determined by the build of the peripheral organ of hearing.

CHAPTER IX

TIME

WHEN two sensations of different temporal positions are given, they make up an experience of at least a greater duration than did either. And when the two are far enough apart temporally, we notice an interval of time between them. When two or more sounds follow one another as in the noise of winding up a clock, we notice at the greatest rates only an irregularity or roughness in the flow of sounds. This we might be tempted to call a rough time-surface; but we do not usually do so; we speak rather of an irregular, interrupted sound. A rough touch implies not only that the area of touch is extended in two dimensions, but that it is also present in a *third* dimension; this, however, is not actually presented to us in touch, but is inferred from the differences of intensity of pressure from point to point of the surface or from the sensation of side-pull exerted upon the skin by the rough surface and felt by *muscular* sensation. In vision we can *see* the roughness of a surface, for the vision of two eyes gives us three dimensions of extension. But time never exceeds one dimension, so that the flow of time can be represented by a straight line.

When the two sounds are separated by not more than 0·44 of a second they appear as members of a unitary group whose parts are not yet separate from one another. Longer intervals strike us as distinct pieces of time. A time of 0·7–0.8 seconds seems to stand before the mind as a single whole. From 0·9 to 2·3 seconds this unity seems to dissolve. We have now time to lose hold of the first sound and to await the second. When we do this most easily and best, we feel that our attention is making its most natural step or span. If a warning signal is to be given for any purpose, it should precede the action required by about one and a half seconds. The time-span may by effort be increased up to about four seconds. Times less than three quarters of a second seem "short," times longer than that "long."

The best time senses are those whose sensations begin and end sharply and fully. This we find in touch, articular and muscular sense, sound and sight. Of these sight is much less efficient than the others. As man is a social animal, and his best means of communication is sound, a strong connexion has been laid down in our nervous system between sound impressions and motor response and between one response and the next. Co-operative work and social arts like dancing strengthen and extend these connexions. Both muscular and articular sensations are involved therein: the muscular to make the movement under the control of the will and the articular to regulate its accuracy. A good rhythm may be made with the lips alone, or, as ordinarily in singing, with the vocal chords. A musical conductor usually beats time silently; and as he himself hardly sees his own movements for watching his players, he must feel that his movements correspond to the divisions of time he feels inwardly and intends to maintain. Dancing, although it is not so patently artistic to the dancer as to the spectator, is for the former much more rhythmical. The sense of sight lacks this neural connexion with muscular response and so is a poor time-sense or vehicle for rhythm, although it allows of very precise temporal regulation. But, though practically inefficient, vision does not seem to lack any of the time and rhythm properties of even so fine a sense as hearing.[1]

When times are longer than four seconds, they can only be estimated by some indirect mental effort. We try to gauge them by the flow of our experiences, by the many or few things we had time to think of, by our impatience at delay, or best of all perhaps by counting inwardly at a known regular rate. We are liable to great errors in estimating long intervals—apart from counting or thinking of a fixed melody at a fixed rate, e.g. a march, or the like—as everyone knows. There is some evidence that long

[1] K. Koffka, *Ztsch. Psych.*, 1909, **52**, 1 ff.

times can be estimated very accurately subconsciously in sleep and in the state of hypnosis.

In rhythm we have the complex forms of time sense. A series of impressions may be noticeably regular, and may even be divided into groups without forming a rhythm. Rhythm requires a special dividing and individualising process, namely, accentuation. Comparison of visual and auditory forms makes this clear. A series of bell-tones at the rate of three per second may seem as regular and continuous as a simple line pattern on glazed tiles. It may not readily fall into parts. Even though it does, however, it may appear no more divided than a complex line pattern. In vision we always feel that rhythm is only metaphorically applicable to such figures. For the illustration of rhythm we need to break a picture into clear parts and to carry the eyes in distant steps from point to point, as from tree to tree in the depth of a landscape, or from rock to tree, cloud, house, stream, back to rock, or the like. Or the line pattern must be broken into larger units by special marks, differing perhaps slightly from one another. Then we feel more inclined to speak of rhythm in visual art as against mere regularity and grouping. So in sounds, where the series may be as little physically subdivided as a simple pattern, complex units or periods can only be completely marked off by accent. Each one then seems to stand by itself, and the time-interval between two, though necessarily there as a felt-time, is nevertheless taken as empty or dead, or as a mere lapse of time between the end of one unit and the beginning of the next. It seems to share to a less extent in the formation of the rhythmic figure than the inner times, although it is, of course, really quite as important. In this respect it resembles the interval between two parts of a melody separated by a cadence ; this is an interval, of course, but it seems dead, without the quickening of an essential relation. And the melody breaks there because the cadence brings the motion to a full or partial close by the unifying fixative power of consonance and tonic or dominant ; the melody is renewed in a new form with the next tone. Rhythms thus form definite periodical figures in a flowing series of presentations.

Rhythms may be objective or subjective. Objective rhythms occur when one sound in each period is made intenser or longer than the others or when the interval following one of the sounds is slightly lengthened. The functions of these factors are not identical or substitutive, however. Intensity has a group-beginning effect, duration a group-ending effect.[1] Pitch also affects rhythm in so far as the higher tone is intrinsically more intense (for the same physical force). But when equal apparent intensity is secured, pitch shows no influence upon rhythm. A rhythm in which the louder, longer [2] or higher pitched sound begins the group, may be changed to one in which that sound ends the group by increasing sufficiently the interval following that sound, and vice versa.[3] Rhythm then appears when one or other of the magnitudes that characterise the parts of the figure is suitably increased.

All these devices are used in music according to the capacities of the instrument being played, e.g. piano or organ. The organ cannot produce differences of intensity quickly enough for the purposes of rhythm. Similar differences are found in the verse of different languages, e.g. French and English, to which Latin and Greek may have been somewhat parallel. French is commonly said to be entirely devoid of stress, all syllables having the same value. Perhaps it would be truer to say that its stresses are not fixed for each word-form as in English and German, but vary with the context of the word and with meaning and emotion. Its poetry has, therefore, a less definite basis for its rhythm than other languages have. Latin was perhaps similar though it seems to have forced itself into the moulds natural to the stressful language of the Greek.

Rhythms are subjective when they appear in sounds or sights that are physically exactly periodic and equal. When we listen to the beats of a perfectly balanced metronome, they may appear for a time to be merely regular;

[1] T. L. Bolton, *Amer. J. Psych.*, 1893, **6**, 145 ff. H. Woodrow, *Psych. Rev.*, 1911, **19**, 54 ff.

[2] As it may on occasion, e.g. by inner effort of accentuation by the subject, etc.

[3] Woodrow, op. cit.

but we cannot hear them for long or with any thought of possible rhythm ere a rhythm appears in them. One sound in every two, three, or four seems louder, or, as we must say, becomes louder than the others. The independence of this from the instrument may be tested by shifting the rhythmic group forward a place, when it will continue with equal insistence. Or instead of our two-beat rhythm we may begin a three- or four-beat rhythm, which will then run on by itself.

In both subjective and objective rhythms, but especially in the former, we feel that we are inwardly active. And so the thought will occur that the accentuation of subjective rhythms, like the changes in illusory forms, is not objective, but is due entirely to our activity or rather is entirely a reflexion of our activity. We think or feel the beat louder because we then inwardly beat harder in some way. From this connexion has arisen a very prevalent feeling that it is almost impossible to say what accent or stress in speech is ; especially whether it is merely intensity or something else, and if the latter what this obscure process is. We shall discuss this problem more fully in connexion with the study of illusory forms. There is undoubtedly an inner activity. That is part and parcel of the fact that rhythm is essentially art, something enjoyed in and for itself. It is almost impossible to get animals to dance because they have not reached the stage of cognitive complexity required for attending to experiences for their own sake. This requires abstraction and therefore highly developed cognition. But there is no reason to suppose that an animal does not hear an objective rhythm with all its intensities, lengths, and times, and the figures they form. We, however, have reached the stage of also attending to these figures, of carrying in our mind a pattern of attitudes of expectation parallel to the rhythmic pattern and of fitting our activity exactly to it. This coincidence makes even *equal* sounds rhythmical. Then they simply *are* rhythmical and share the nature of objective rhythms. As objective rhythm includes intenser and longer sounds and longer times, so may the subjective rhythm too. These factors will probably appear in subjective rhythms according to the perceptual habits of the auditor, e.g. if he is more accustomed to length than intensity accents, etc. Possibly the use of intensity for accentuation predominates in all of us owing to the strong habits of our speech and other motor rhythms. Observations under incognitive procedure point to this predominance.[1] But, of course, when keen observation is turned upon illusory accents, they will disappear, as the subjective accentuation is then eliminated by concentration upon the objective constants. Though the agent be subjective, the phenomena of all rhythms (like difference-tones) are essentially objective or properties of the sense-data that compose the rhythmic figure. This conclusion points, not to a mysterious subjective source of illusion or of stress, but to the ultimately sensory origin of the patterns of our subjective activity in this case. Our attentional processes, in other words, are probably an outgrowth of our sensory ones, even although they are reflexly applied to them. It seems only thus that we may hope to explain the origin and more especially the alterative power of attention on sensory complexes.

This is supported by the carefully proved fact that rhythm is inherent in the sensory complex of sounds, or light-flashes or touches, etc., which it characterises, no matter what processes from other senses may accompany it. The swings and movements of body, feet or head that rhythm evokes are not its cause. Rather are they the natural outcome of the activity of attention so characteristic of rhythmic experiences. Nor do we need to derive rhythm from the rhythmic functions apparent in reflex actions. If the nervous system has invented a mechanism to produce rhythm in reflexes, why should it not have bred one for the special use of its higher regions, so that we may have rhythms moulded directly into any suitable forms of experience?

A strong rhythm arouses us, we act inwardly to it, and this activity in turn flows through its well-established channels into muscular movements. For we have made these movements often to the accompaniment of this same typical activity even apart from the rhythm just given.

[1] E. Meumann, *Phil. Stud.*, 1894, **10**, 249 ff., 393 ff.; 1896, **12**, 127 ff.

Thus in order the better to observe and to learn rhythms, we often carry out some accustomed more or less rhythmic activity while the new impressions are being given—we count, tap, nod the head, say tick-tock, etc. This is only a method, not a necessary means of learning. Rapid and probably best progress can be made by listening to different rhythms in turn and by comparing and describing them. The mind then certainly is turned upon the end required instead of possibly never passing from the intended counting to the hearing and intention of rhythm.

The number of beats per group in a subjective rhythm generally varies with their rate of succession, increasing with the faster rates. But the character of each rhythm, e.g. the greater vividness of twos, modifies this rule somewhat. The combination that is generally most pleasing makes the product of the time between two beats and the number of them average somewhat over one second.[1] The limits for lengths of time between beats varies from one tenth (*ibid.*) to 2·4 seconds.[2] Sound rhythms lie towards shorter times than do visual rhythms (which do not occur below 0·3 sec. and favour rates from 0·75 to 1·5 seconds between beats. The lengths of visual periods extend from 0·65 to 5·6 seconds). The largest periods are formed when smaller groups are grouped together with a specially strong accent once in the whole period. Long periods are generally characterised by accents of different degrees. These accents serve to bind a series of times together into a group that otherwise would be too long for the time-sense to apprehend in a unity. Subjective activity thus helps to extend the natural spontaneous range of integration.

Though rhythms of two, three, and four units, simple or compound, are the easiest, others of five or seven or more beats are readily produced, both objectively and subjectively. Usually so easy to hear in an objective form, they are often surprisingly hard to maintain subjectively in connexion with a series of perfectly equal beats. But practice readily makes the process almost automatic. A rhythm of five or of seven must be distinguished from an

[1] Bolton, op. cit., 214 ff.
[2] Koffka, op. cit.

alternating rhythm of two and three, or of three and four, such as we find in Brahms' Hungarian Variations. The difficulty of these odd-numbered rhythms has kept them out of music for the most part, but modern music affords examples, e.g. Tchaikovsky's Pathetic Symphony, 2nd movement, Chopin's Sonata in C minor, opus 41. And recent music is rapidly expanding its powers of rhythmical freedom and complication. To have command of a rhythm you must be able to keep it up indefinitely and unfailingly apart from all such accompaniments or substitutes as counting. It must be secure in your mind, as are the words of a familiar recitation or a dance form. Our ability to keep up the same rhythm in spite of changes of speed shows us the same sense of proportion as we noticed in dealing with systemic forms.

The music of primitive peoples often displays a complexity of rhythm that strains or even baffles the rhythmic capacity of the European musician. Probably our music devotes so much attention to melodic and harmonic form that its rhythmic development has hitherto remained comparatively simple. The most rhythmic of western music—Hungarian, Negro, Scotch (bagpipe) is either very simple in harmony or almost devoid of it.

CHAPTER X

ILLUSORY MODIFICATIONS OF FORM

WHEN we put several lines together to form a figure, they seem in most cases to have no effect upon one another. They lie side by side, merely forming a whole in which each appears exactly as it does in isolation. But grouping sometimes alters lines in a very noticeable way, and closer examinations show that slight modifications frequently occur. These changes of appearances are called illusions. They appertain to the chief features of form—to the size and straightness or direction of distances, lines, and masses.

Some distortions are due to external physical causes. A familiar example is the stick that appears bent in water. Such effects are of no psychological interest, for we then see exactly what the eye sees. And so we may expect to

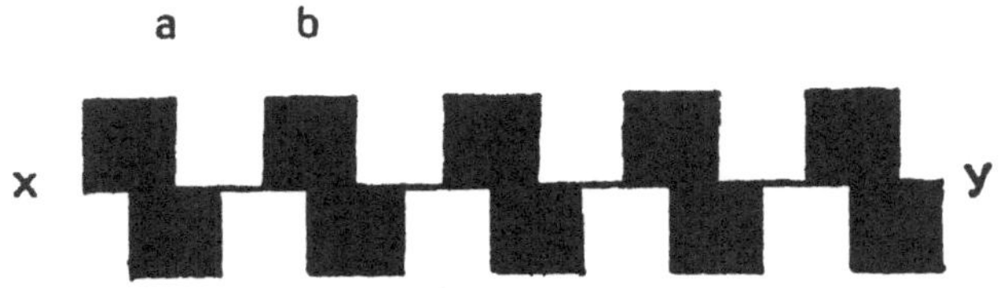

FIG. 12.

find a class of illusions caused by physical changes within the eye. Illusions of irradiation seem to be such. A black square on a white ground looks smaller than an equal white square on black. The vigorous process of white on the retina may be supposed to overflow the precise boundary given to it by the light that strikes the eye. It " radiates " into the feebler process of black, a process that seems to be due not so much to stimulation as to recovery or rest from stimulation. This class of illusion still stands outside the circle of interest of pure psychology. It tells us nothing about the influence of experiences upon one another.

Irradiation is largely, if not wholly, responsible for a number of illusions of direction. When as in Fig. 12 a white corner borders on a black area, the white overflows a little into the black. The white corner below *a* in Fig. 12 lies not only a little to the left of the point of the black corner at *a* that is really directly above it, but also a little lower. Similarly the white corner below *b* lies for the eye rather to the right and above its real position. These alternate downwards and upwards shifts are less noticeable in isolation than in the figure, because their effect is then cumulative in the line *x–y*. There seems to be a distinct slope up from *x* to *y*. If the figure is inverted, the opposite deflection will be seen. If it is made in such a form as to allow of sliding the upper half (above *x–y*) to and fro over the lower half, the central boundary *x–y* will seem to slope alternately one way and the other. Compare Hering's figures and Poggendorff's figure (Fig. 13).

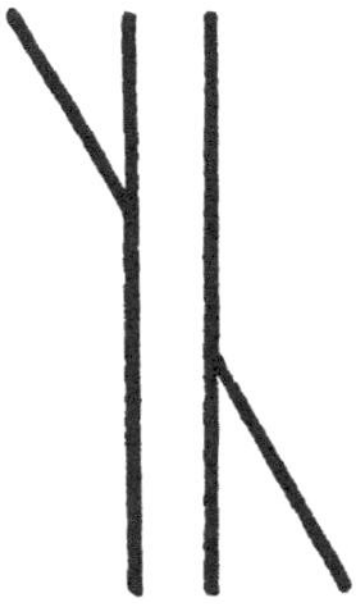

FIG. 13.

Psychologically purest are the illusions of size. They seem to embody changes (in the features of sensations) that have no detectable physical or physiological causes. And it is perhaps inevitable that these illusions should be confined to the feature of size. For size is the only primary and variant feature of distance (which we have recognised as the element of form). The Müller-Lyer figure gives the most striking illusion of form. No cause for the apparent shortening of the horizontal line in A or for the lengthening of the same line in B (Fig. 14) has yet been established that operates either within the eye (or the retina) or outside of it. Nor does any such peripheral cause seem probable. The one most persistently alleged is the movements made by the eyes in inspection of the figure. But even if these movements were exactly equivalent to the apparent length of the lines, which they are far from being, we might still properly claim that the eye movements followed the sizes apparent to vision. For why should the eyes take it upon themselves to move in any fixed way except at the instigation of what is seen? And the illusion persists when the eye sharply and steadily fixates any point of the figure or when the figure is exposed for so short a time that eye movements are impossible. If the two figures are projected alternately upon a screen so that their middle lines coincide, this middle line is seen to shorten

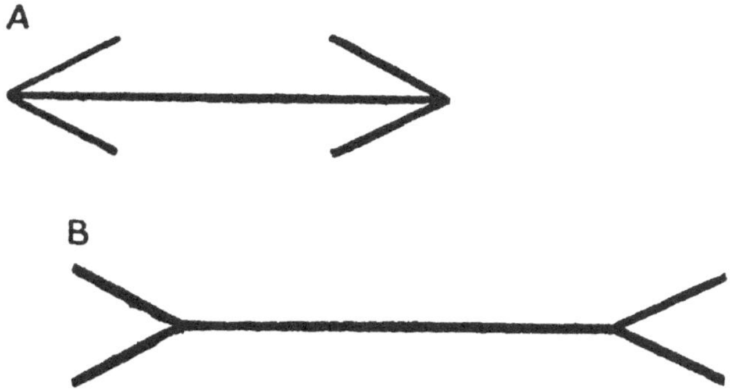

FIG. 14.

and lengthen as if its ends were moving. This holds for any orientation of the figure to the observer. It is best for a certain rate of alternation (3 or 4 per second).

Careful observation during the illusion shows that the prominent feature of it is the space occupied by the figure as a whole, more or less. Our judgments are always greatly influenced by this total space. If we are to be strict in our reference to the horizontal line, we must exert ourselves to break up the figure and to concentrate on the part specified. Weakening of the side lines in thickness or colour, and strengthening of the middle line make this analysis easier. The abstraction may also be cultivated by practice until the illusion even disappears entirely. Some people of primitive culture naturally incline to this analytic attitude.

A circle in the midst of larger circles looks smaller than when it is surrounded by circles smaller than itself. The circles do not join together to form a unitary figure, but we look at each one as a separate thing surrounded by others as distinct. The apparent change of direction in the two parts of the sloping line in Poggendorff's figure (Fig. 13) may partly be due to this cause. Each of its groups of three lines above and below seems to form a separate part of the whole and so the break in the middle looks larger than it really is. If the parallel lines are lengthened or set farther apart, the illusion increases, probably because they then draw the attention into the vertical direction and upon the two parts. If the cross-line is lengthened, the illusion decreases, because the greater obtrusiveness of that line then emphasises it and its unity. A row of dots seems to give a greater distance than the unfilled distance between the two outer dots. Momentary exposure gives the greatest illusory effect. But if there is only one dot (or two) in the space, the divided lengths seem shorter. Here again we are led away by the comparable shortness of the lengths given by division.

For some obscure reason a horizontal line seems shorter than an equal vertical one. For more obvious reasons the extent of a surface is overestimated as compared with a line. The dimensions of the surface of a solid object, such as a cube or cylinder, are overestimated as compared with lines or surfaces. And the length of a cylinder is overestimated as against its diameter. "In the case of the area illusions it is a vague feeling of 'more of it' with reference to the area as compared with the line; and in the case of the volume illusion, it is a vague notion of 'more of it' with reference to the surface of the solid as compared with a mere surface, which leads to the overestimation." [1]

The student who is specially interested in visual form should make a careful study of these and other similar illusions. For such motives enter extensively into the work of art, ornamentation, pictures, dress fabrics, and the like. In fact, the basis of many of the special effects of composition is essentially of the same kind. The artist often heightens them by supplementary motives, while he inserts others which will prevent the observer from discovering the primary means towards the special effect. "Ars est celare artem" is a proverb that greatly exaggerates the importance of this procedure in art.

Some of the illusions, e.g. the Müller-Lyer figure, the filled and empty distance, probably occur in the sense of

[1] Seashore, *Psychology in Daily Life.* New York, 1914, p. 172.

touch. But for obvious reasons they are not nearly so pronounced or noticeable. In the other two senses of form there are at the most only traces of them.

There are, of course, also illusions that have nothing to do with form. A notable example is that of weight. The weight of an object is affected by the extension of the arm (directly), by the tightness of one's grasp of it (inversely), by the size of the skin area in contact with it (inversely), by the weight of the object lifted before it (inversely), by the warmth or coldness of it (directly), by the weight its appearance suggests (inversely), by the apparent size of it (inversely), and by the distinctness of its apparent size (inversely). Some of these effects can be traced to peripheral causes, some are due to contrast between the strain expected or the force applied and the strain actually felt, and some are due to mistaken references. In accordance therewith it is found that the illusion " remains undiminished and tends to grow more constant with long continued practice so long as the observer is not aware of its existence " ; that " the force of the illusion is decreased when its existence becomes known or suspected " ; but that " the illusion can perhaps never be eradicated by practice " ; that " one soon learns to make conscious allowance for it " ; and that " there is a general tendency to make allowance for it unconsciously " (op. cit., 175 ff.).

Illusions that can appear in a single dimension of vision, e.g. that of filled and empty space, can be detected also with similar arrangements of time-intervals.

We are still unable to give a final theory of the psychological illusions. If we consider physical causes as definitely excluded, there are three possibilities. (1) The illusions are due to the interaction of sensory units such as distances, lines, figures, amongst one another. They would represent the dynamics of sense-data, as it were. (2) They are due to, and reside in, the processes of judgment that comparison of such sensory magnitudes necessarily implies. We fail to see their exact relative values because of the foggy atmosphere of cognition that lies between us and them. (3) They are due to the interaction of sensory magnitudes and subjective attitudes, syntheses of attention, and the like. The prevalent tendency has always been to refer illusions either to purely external causes and physical " errors of vision " or to the purely subjective distortions of judgment. Units of sensation are commonly supposed to lie inert beside one another without mutual interference.

The source in judgment (2) seems acceptable since cognition is otherwise often at fault. Even in pure logic errors are common ; but they can be corrected by a little attention, whereas illusions require much practice. Again, the gradual annulment of the illusion by practice suggests that the fog of misdirected attention (with its special effects) has then merely rolled away leaving us in direct contact with the sensory data. But if the source of the illusion lies in the process of judgment alone, no positive effect can have rolled away. We have merely brought our estimation of the relative sizes of the lines into parallel with their relative physical sizes. The illusions consist not in putting something where there was nothing, but in altering the magnitudes of distances and lines from those values they have when they are dependent solely upon the simplest sensory stimulus, as shown in a single standard line. So judgment is not the only process involved.

On the contrary, it is tempting to think that there is no fog in cognition at all, but that the units of experience interact with one another like the units of matter. There must surely be some sort of purely mental dynamics. The analysis of mind that has hitherto been attained on the assumption that its units form an inert aggregate, is far from satisfactory. But a positive hypothesis to the contrary requires the most exact and systematic foundations. The fragmentary effects found in illusions hardly provide a broad enough basis for it.

So we seem urged towards the third alternative that their cause is the interaction of subjective, perceptual and other attitudes with the sensory complexes of the figures. Why this interaction should make sensory magnitudes look larger or smaller than they " really " are, is by no means clear. For the alteration must surely be considered to be a strong positive effect, not merely an " illusion." Illusory effects are physically unreal, of course. But, as within the mind, they must surely be considered real :

i.e. the sensory magnitudes are really altered in themselves, as experiences. The whole space of the Müller-Lyer figure makes the horizontal line (not look, but be) larger or smaller. This change cannot well have been *transported* from the subjective group of forces into the sensory group. It must rather be that in a mind highly cultivated in cognitive observation these higher processes, though ultimately based upon the sensory ones, yet finally react upon them and modify them. How they do so is by no means clear.

One line of solution seems definitely excluded. We cannot reconsider the older view that sensory distances and intervals and other such integrates are entirely products of the reason working upon some obscure data of sense that possess only quality and intensity. Attributes of position and extent, both systemic and temporal, and integrates of distance, etc., must be recognised as facts independent of the higher reaches of cognition—indeed, as facts by which higher cognition itself becomes possible and is filled.

CHAPTER XI

MOTION

THE experience of motion may be said to be a compound involving differences in both systemic and temporal position. This does not mean that in a short motion we can distinguish separately from one another all the positions implicitly involved in it, any more than in a tone's volume we can pick out all the particles of sound we are entitled to suppose it contains, or than in a big extent of warmth we can count all the particles of warmth that we could elicit by careful examination from the area of skin warmed. In a continuous motion all such positional differences are more or less evenly graded in a unity. But they are there to mark the boundaries of motion, to define its position as a whole and to determine its speed. Speed is a function of distance traversed and time spent in the motion ; but in apprehending a motion psychologically we do not need to have apprehended these factors separately or explicitly. What we primarily apprehend is the motion and its speed, which can be compared as an unanalysed unity with any another similar speed and motion.

The senses of motion will, of course, be those that give distance and form well, since all the senses give temporal positions well enough for the purpose. So the best motion-senses are vision, articular sense, touch and hearing. And all circumstances improve motion that improve its formal and temporal bases. This seems to be the reason why mere motion apparently forces us to attend to it, and the more strongly in proportion to its speed. The moving stimulus is not yet subject to adaptation and diffusion into the surrounding area. Rapid illumination similarly favours apprehension of form.

A striking feature of motion is met with in vision. This seems rather to concern the physiological process underlying motion than any mental process dealing with its apprehension. It is now familiar to everyone in the cinematograph, which throws on the screen a rapid series of pictures. None of these contains any motion at all; each is merely an instantaneous photograph of a phase of the scene. Nor does the single picture move as a whole, for the change from picture to picture is accomplished during a dark interval in which the light of the lantern is cut off by a sector of a rotating disc. Under the proper conditions of operation we do not notice any discontinuity or flicker corresponding to these light and dark phases. But the series of instantaneous photographs thus thrown on the screen merges into a continuous view of moving objects. Each picture represents a phase of the motion which is separated by a gap from the preceding and following phases; but the series as a sequence gives us the whole motion without any gaps. The brain, so we must suppose, is able to do without the missing fragments.

This may be roughly explained by reference to Fig. 6 (p. 66). The stimuli *a* and *b*, which are separated by a little distance on the field of receptors, are now given consecutively after a certain regular interval of time. But the sensation B does not appear in its maximal strength suddenly; it only gradually reaches the maximum for any strength of stimulus; and it will not reach even that maximum if the time of application of the stimulus is too short. Similarly sensation A does not disappear immediately on the removal of the stimulus; it merely begins to fade down from the maximum it had attained. Therefore under suitable conditions the increasing sensation B will "meet" and partially overlap the decreasing sensation A; and the summation of the overlapping parts will make sensation A run smoothly into sensation B. But as B is still increasing, it will appear to be the point at which the stimulus actually is situated at the moment. Similarly for sensations B and C, etc. Therefore, under favourable conditions the sequence of A B C D E F, etc., sensations, excited from points on the periphery that are separated by considerable spaces, must be equivalent in continuity to the continuous sensation streak A–F etc., produced by moving a stimulus continuously over the field of receptors between the first and last points of application.

The only difference will be that for the same intensity of stimulus in the two cases (discrete and continuous), the latter will give the more intense sensation. For the overlapping is then not only deeper, but the points of application follow more quickly, so that the first spot of sensation has less time for decrease ere the second appears. So in the cinema picture we find that the brightness decreases with the increase of the obscuration time—according to Talbot's law; $\frac{W^\circ\, I(w)+I(b)B^\circ}{W^\circ+B^\circ}=I(g)$, where W° and B° are the angular extents of the black and white phases, and I(w), I(b) and I(g) are the relative intensities of the white and black phases and of the resultant fused intensity (grey).[1]

It is also clear that the nearer together the stimuli *a* and *b* are set, the longer may be the time interval between them without any break in the continuity of resulting motion. There is then a greater height of serviceable overlapping of sensation spots; i.e. it will be longer before the spot has died down too far for any continuity by overlapping to be attained in the sequence of spots. Similarly when the time interval is reduced, the component spots may be farther apart for optimal movement. Other variable factors may be readily imagined. The subject has been treated mathematically by Koffka.[2] The fundamental object of study in experimental work on such "stroboscopic" motion consists of two points of light or two positions of a simple figure, instead of the series given in the cinematograph. It is advisable to rid the experimental conditions of the perceptual ideas and expectations

[1] The fusion of the black and white phases referred to in Talbot's law is also affected favourably by increase in the difference of the duration of the phases, by decrease in the difference of their brightness, and by increase in their mean brightness (cf. Weber's law). These relations can also be explained by reference to the relations of overlapping contacts. Greater brightness is the analogue of greater intensity, and longer duration becomes greater relative intensity owing to the gradual increase of excitation in the first moments.

[2] *Ztsch. Psych.*, 1919, **82**, 25 ff.

of movement that familiar objects in motion excite, making nonsense syllables of motion, as it were. Such expectations are found to be forceful causes, so that a disc shown at the eight corners of an octagon will appear to move along the sides of this figure, whereas if the octagon is surrounded by a larger circle the disc will seem to roll round it as if it were running in a circular grove.[1] Similarly a line sloping up from the middle point of another one at an acute angle will seem to fall into the horizontal line through the shorter distance on successive presentation of the lines; but if the angle is gradually increased till it is greater than a right angle, it will "fall" through the large angle, instead of through the smaller one in the opposite direction.

Beyond the conditions for optimal movement partial or at least very evanescent, hardly detectable, movements occur, as if the light shown in a series of positions seemed to pass behind a paling in which the laths were of gradually larger size until there was hardly space left for the light to shine through. At the least there is only a tremor of each light—in the direction of successive illumination—as it glows up.

Serious criticism of this theory of motion by overlapping central resultants has been given by F. Hillebrand,[2] who prefers to connect the facts with certain positional phenomena of vision that are very familiar. When we fixate a point straight ahead, its image falls on the fovea; when we look some distance to the right, the image of the point fixated again falls on the fovea, but the point now seems to be far to the right of the point first fixated; and neither point appears to have moved, although the first total image was shifted over the retina to the right. Nothing, however, is perceived during this rapid change of fixation, so that there is no effectual gliding of a stimulus over the retina, but only two successive stationary stimulations, brought into connexion by the complex processes of perception. Identification of the two depends upon the presence of a common part; something is added on at the right in place of what lapses from sight on the left. We are practically unaware of the movements of the eyes, except in so far as

[1] Cf. Linke, *Psych. St.*, **3**, p. 524.
[2] *Ztsch. Psych.*, 1922, **89**, 209 ff; **90**, 1 ff.

we intend them, so that the " revaluation " of the foveal position with reference to our body is " central," not a product of sensory integration (e.g. vision plus eye-muscular sensation). When we intend no eye-movement and make none, any retinal displacement due to motion of objects or forced motion of the eyeball is taken as external motion of what is seen. If the intended eye-movement does not take place, as in states of paralysis, the objects of vision also seem to move, although they have not been displaced on the retina at all. For they would have been displaced, had the eye really moved as intended and, to bring them then to their first place on the retina, they would have had to be moved by an equivalent amount in the opposite direction: therefore, as the eye did not move, the " patient " perceives this unexpected or unintended " movement " as a real one. In states of partial paralysis of the eye-muscles, the objects of vision seem to move to the extent required by the paralysis: for the remainder they remain still as in a normal eye-movement of that actual amount. Contrariwise when we follow a rapid movement with the eye we change our fixation to keep pace with it and so we see the movement as objectively as when we watch it with unaltered fixation, in spite of the gaps in our perception. Stroboscopic motion displays great perceptual freedom: it appears even when we give " a plant, a bird-cage, and a bunch of grapes " in succession, so that it rather points to some independent " central " factor than to the overlapping of the immediate central resultants of peripheral excitation.

In order to carry these processes of positional revaluation into the sphere of stroboscopic motion, Hillebrand requires only to postulate a *gradual* revaluation in order to account for the time factor and to explain its anomalies. As an example of anomaly we need only cite the fact that the optimal motion may persist even for negative time-intervals, i.e. when presentation 2 slightly precedes No. 1. But, however attractive Hillebrand's theory may be, it has serious difficulties to face, e.g. the presence of many simultaneous movements as in many complex figure film-displays. We cannot feel attracted to the view that observers really see only one movement—the one they follow, and that all the others are illusory in a secondary sense, illusory illusions, "supposed reminiscences."

The whole matter is evidently extremely complex in fact, and unclear in theory, however precise it may all be for practice such as the cinema implies. The facts of stroboscopic movement too seem themselves to be duplex. Dimmick[1] was able to confirm them under an instruction "to characterise the perception or to state its meaning," but found that they disappeared under the instruction "to report in strictly psychological terms upon the processes experienced," when a flash was always reported, extending in optimal motion from the first real component (a line) to the second, in partial movements only part of the way. Coloured stimuli did not alter the grey, but increase of brightness decreased its brightness. There was no movement in the grey flash. We may perhaps compare this destruction of motion with the effect of staring at stereoscopic pictures, when the solidity disappears. We do not therefore infer that there was no solidity in the ordinary process of inspection or that solidity is only a "meaning" or a "perception," unless we mean by the latter terms just such things as solidity. Neither solidity nor motion may be eviscerated by classifying it as "meaning" or "alleged reminiscence," etc. We may therefore hold to the psychical reality of motion, whatever its basis may be. The term integration best recognises both its psychical substance, as it were, its primary objectivity in sense, in relation to differences of position, and prior to central processes of attention, and its later fluidity and mobility, when equivalent bases of positional differences are produced by the complications of sense. Our chief task at the present stage of psychology is to get the chief facts of various regions of sense and its integrations into good systematic order when the status of such complexities may become clearer. And cinematic motion appears in various senses, even when there is no such thing as change of fixation and intentional movement of the organ.

In hearing the subtle motion that results in this way is of great importance. It is the essence of melody, the bond that unites a series of tones of steady unwavering pitch.

[1] *Amer. J. Psych.*, 1920, **31**, 317 ff.

Here again we find that the "illusion" of motion is the stronger the smaller the interval between successive tones. "Conjunct" motion is best for melody, as musicians say. There is surprising regularity in the frequencies with which the various intervals are used in melodies. The larger the interval in question, the less often is it used proportionately; and for very different types of music—primitive and modern European, Asiatic European and American (Indian)—the proportion of decrease appears to be 60 per cent for every extra semitone from the minor second to the octave. It seems doubtful on careful consideration whether the consonant intervals really alter this proportion appreciably by increasing the frequency, as at first glance they seem to do and as musicians say they do. For some unknown reason an interval is used proportionately oftener for a melodic descent than for ascent, the smaller it is.[1]

When two melodies are to be sounded simultaneously, the art of music consists in making them run easily together without disturbing one another's flow. This disturbance comes most of all from the "perfect" consonances and dissonances, which create a loss of distinction of the tones of either melody (by their too great unity and by their confusion respectively). So we find that special precautions have to be taken in approaching either a consonance or a dissonance, especially the former, and in leaving a dissonance (because it *must* be left). Consonances may be approached by "contrary motion," both the previous tones of either melody (or "voice") lying either within the interval of the consonance or without it. A dissonance may be approached by "preparation," i.e. by holding on as one of its tones the tone preceding it in the same voice; the other one is then freed from confusion with it; or, as in the most "modern" music, by using "step" of a semitone or tone instead of this repetition of the same tone: modern ears are practised and skilled, and so can do more than was usually done in earlier music, although the kind of thing done is psychologically the

[1] Cf. H. J. Watt, *The Functions of the Size of Intervals in Melodies*. *Br. J. Psych.*, 1924, **14**, 370 ff. Also *Melody, Music and Letters*, 1924, **5**, 272 ff.

same. Obviously, two identical consonances or dissonances (of the same interval) on different notes of the scale after one another would be a great disturbance of melodic flow; for the second would be approached by similar motion even if the first one had been successfully negotiated.

The putting of several melodies or voices together is not a different task from two-part writing; it is only a step further in the same work. And its problems are the same, except that the larger number of voices makes the mutually disturbing effect of any two less noticeable. Rules are therefore the more relaxed in part writing the greater the number of parts. Of a number of parts the lowest is the most noticeable, the highest next and the inner ones less. So the most care has to be given to the mutual relation of the outside parts, next most to that of the lowest and a higher part, next to that of highest and a lower part, while the middle parts require least care.

Thus we see how the laws of part-writing and composition follow from the psychological nature of our sensations of hearing. Chords are typical incidents in the flow of three or four or more parts and the laws of their "resolution" are formulæ for the melodic movements of their parts, the rule being that the difficult or dissonant notes of a discord shall move, as usual in all good melody, by as short steps as possible, while the other notes move so as to avoid creating disturbances of melodic flow on their own part, i.e. they are free to do as they like provided they do it inoffensively.

The cinematic process of movement has been experimentally verified for the sense of touch.[1] Under certain conditions of time, distance, and intensity an optimal impression of movement from one point to the other occurs in the direction of actual succession. The longer the stimulus the relatively shorter must the time-interval be; this may be due to the lowering and narrowing of intensity by adaptation. The greater the distance between the stimuli, the greater must the time interval be; i.e. to obtain an optimal movement between distant stimuli, the mound of excitation of the first must be allowed to fall low till it runs evenly into the other. The greater the distance

[1] H. E. Burtt, *J. Exper. Psych.*, 1917, **2**, 371 ff.

between the stimuli, the greater the intensity required; the greater intensity will spread the mound farther out around. The greater the intensity, the less must the time-interval be; possibly the greater intensity falls off more rapidly at first. Finally, if the intensity of the second is greater than that of the first, the illusory movement is sometimes produced in the reverse direction; this must be connected with the swifter entry of a greater stimulus, so that upon favourable occasion the second stimulus is centrally first. Evidently all these rules and phenomena are reducible to functions of the central physiological forces of excitation underlying the temporal sequence of events. They confirm our hypothesis that all the senses are constituted and function after the same pattern. And the hypothesis of psychophysical parallelism is thereby carried a stage further.

When a visual motion, e.g. a flowing river, has been observed for some little time and the eye is turned away from it, the surface then looked at shows an illusory movement in the opposite direction. The direction of the after-motion is always the projected contrary of that produced in the retina by the moving object. The after-motion is in every way a true visual motion, although its object is illusory. It can be quite obtrusive or real-like or it can be so unobtrusive as to be almost imaginary. These differences it shares with cinematic motions. Its cause is evidently physiological and cerebral, but it has not yet been satisfactorily formulated. The after-motion has also been demonstrated in the sense of touch.[1]

These and other facts keep insistently alive the view that motion is a sensational element in no way integrated from simpler sensory particles. Motion, like distance and extent, can be observed even while its direction is undetectable. But in this respect motion is far more obtrusive than distance and extent are. As already noted at the beginning of the chapter, however, none of these facts need prevent us referring motion to an integration of minimal particles differing in systemic and temporal position, for we do not require to distinguish these separately at all in such a process. Nor do we need to have detail and definition

[1] W. A. Thalman, *Amer. J. Psych.*, 1922, **33**, 268 ff.

enough for the perception of direction. It is even possible, as it seems a fact, that in unusual circumstances of vision, motion may be detectable when nothing else can be seen at all.[1] Conditions very similar to this normally exist on the periphery of the field of vision. The status we have given to motion implies merely that if static details were visible (i.e. distinguishable) the first seen motion would take its place amongst them without any processes of inference. Its constituent particles, earliest visible as mere motion, would now be the constituent particles of forms in motion (or devoid of motion as the case might be). The motion would not have to be experimentally or inferentially connected with them apart from any such sensory identity.

As already noticed in Chapter X, motions are produced when different aspects of an illusory figure, e.g. the Müller-Lyer, are given alternately in succession. So long as the synthetic attitude of observation required by the illusion is maintained, the motion persists as if it were real. Evidently the illusory changes are real enough to create motions between them, however dependent they are on subjective conditions. It is also one of the peculiarities of a figure as against its ground that formative movements of expansion outwards take place when it is suddenly and briefly exposed to an eye prepared to see it. These movements stop with a jerk at the boundary of the figure. Similar movements appear when an area in a dark field (e.g. a window seen from outside at night) is suddenly lit or darkened. When ground and figure interchange, as they readily do when they are similar or when both constitute a clear figure, then what before was ground and is now figure alone shows the formative movements. The conditions of attention implied in the apprehension of figure no doubt produce a progressive rapid observation of area from the point of fixation outwards to the boundaries, from which a movement results. As we have seen, it is difficult to hold the balance between objectivity (movement in the sensory process as its conformation rapidly proceeds) and subjectivity (movement due to the rapid progress of attention over positions more or less simultaneously presented).

[1] G. Riddoch, *Brain*, 1917, **40**, 15 ff.

The apprehension of movement depends greatly upon the perceptual processes that accompany, and rest upon it. When we are looking at a point of weak light in the darkness, we often find it difficult to distinguish objective movements from subjective movements that are due to slow progressive movements of the eyes ; but as soon as the light is strong enough to illumine the room, we are no longer in doubt. In such circumstances the perception of movement requires a system of reference and depends upon it. So if we look at a fixed point while observing a moving object, it will seem to move twice as fast as when we follow the moving object with our eyes. For in the former case all motion is attributed to the moving object, but in the latter case half of it is attributed to the moving object and half to the background that is taken to be moving in the opposite direction, each therefore moving half as fast as the total relative motion.[1]

[1] W. Filehne, *Ztsch. Sinnesphys.*, 1921, **53**, 134 ff.

CHAPTER XII

BINAURAL POSITION

WE have now studied all the integrations that are to be found in any single sensory field and that do not directly or indirectly rest upon or involve the use of any other sensory field at the same time. These fields consist of a group of elementary specialised organs of the same kind, spread over a surface, each giving its own particle or " spot " of sensation. The next striking complication of sense is the duplication of such fields of the same kind. Vision and hearing offer obvious instances of this. And there is an " olfactory region " in each half of the nasal cavity.

These smell areas do not seem to add in any way to the variation of positional or extensive aspects of smells. They seem rather in some way to improve the apprehension of sensory quality. But very little is yet known about their functions. It will be for experimental study to discover what minute traces there may be in them of a " dirhinal " integration, hitherto undetected ; or, as it may be, to find this integration already active in some familiar process of smell.

It is the work of the two eyes that raises the duplication of sensory fields to the status of a distinct integrative function. Here we get one of the best instances of the new phase that integration adds to the experiences it unites. In binocular vision the two fields are unified to one field, and the binocular part of this greater area now presents us with a third dimension of vision, which, under exactly similar conditions, either field separately is unable to provide. We shall deal with vision later by itself.

The work of the two ears is by contrast relatively simple. Our knowledge of binaural functions is increasing rapidly at present: and many new facts have not yet been adequately reduced to their most elementary and fundamental components or processes. But it is still true, as until recently it seemed sufficient, to say that the two ears serve a very simple function, one that in the other senses is usually satisfied within the single field of two dimensions. Each ear seems to work in conjunction with the other as if it were an elementary "spot"; so that the two ears form together an extremely limited "field," which then is functionally as single as any special area of touch or vision. Its only remarkable difference is the greater physical distance that separates the component organs of it. This very simple theory of binaural hearing satisfies a large number of the facts; and it therefore offers us a means of arranging them and of gauging their requirements.

The field of the single ear is a peculiar structure. It is a long column of some 16,000 nerve endings that lie along the basilar membrane, near the inside of the outer edge of the whorls of the cochlea. The breadth of it includes only some three to five receptors, the length is therefore some 4000. Now all the functions of hearing that we may call musical, including the apprehension of noise, we have already analysed into a long series of finely differentiated positions (or pitches), each one attributive to a small particle or spot of sound sensation. Music we may therefore regard as a function of one dimension only. And the physiological study of the ear makes it indubitable that this dimension corresponds to the long anatomical one. What about the other very short anatomical dimension, then? Is it used for any purpose?

In the single ear it really seems to have no distinct use, unless it be to give sounds a little breadth as well as length of volume. For although we do right to ignore this "transverse" aspect of the auditory field in considering its longitudinal or musical aspect, we must not forget that a volume having length without some breadth would be nothing at all. But it is of no consequence for the musical nature of sounds that they have little breadth. Only in so far as they vary longitudinally, have they any musical function. Thus by virtue of the abstractive power of the mind musical sounds are independent of their breadth.

But the combined use of the two ears would make this transverse aspect useful, as we may understand by reference to Fig. 6 (p. 66). The stimulation of either ear we may suppose produces a mound of excitation or a sensation that—in respect of its transverse aspect—corresponds to A or B of the figure. This excitation is itself a compound, of course. But it is easy to see that in a certain arrangement the " spots " produced by a few nerve terminals will seem to form a single well-graded spot like A or B. And as the nerve terminals of hearing are arranged brickwise in the transverse aspect, the three to five rows really reduce for this purpose to two to three rows. We may suppose further that the mounds for either ear overlap when they occur together so as to give a final binaural mound of excitation or a small breadth of sensation, most intense in the middle and evenly graded towards its edges. This will be the result when the two ears contribute equal amounts of excitation. When one ear is stimulated much more than the other, its contribution will be correspondingly larger and the maximal point of the resultant will lie towards the side of the stronger contribution, i.e. towards that ear. By suitable variation of the intensities of the components the maximum could be made to shift from one extreme to the other. It matters not in the least to this hypothesis that the two ears lie so much farther apart in the head than any two contacts that feel as one, even on the dullest parts of the skin. Their brain connexions may still be as close together as if the ears were only a quarter of an inch apart. The separation of the organs will merely allow of their being stimulated by the same source of sound with different intensity according to its position relatively to them. And the ears lie on opposite sides of the head so as to make this difference as great as possible.

Such is the skeleton of the psychological or psychophysical theory of binaural hearing that our previous study of hearing suggests as most probable. Let us now consider how it agrees with the physical facts and with the results of experiments on binaural position.

First some details regarding the binaural sensation. This sound ought not only to seem broader than the uniaural one, but also fuller and clearer. For each ear, like each eye, will render some of the musical details better than the other. And yet, of course, the sound should seem much the same musically to either ear. The transverse aspect of the binaural field should also consist of a central binaural part with a uniaural part on either side of this. But only when the uniaural components differ considerably in pitch will these three parts be distinguishable. A higher-pitched tone in the left ear will give a leftward maximum at one point of the length, a lower tone in the right ear a rightwards maximum at another point. And when these two tones lie close enough together in pitch a central part may also be distinguishable. Finally the binaural resultant may vary in intensity as a whole. All these deductions from our hypothesis have been confirmed by careful psychological observation.

We should further infer that the primary differentiation of binaural position consists solely of a single series of a problematical number of just noticeable differences: but not of a circle or sphere of positions. This deduction is more difficult to verify, although it agrees with what has been for some time thought to be the primary variation of binaural hearing. It requires very careful consideration.

The stimulus that a constant source of sound exerts upon the one ear may differ from that upon the other in two ways only: in relative intensity and in phase. The physical intensity of sound varies (ideally) inversely as the square of the distance of the sounding body from the ear. So when this body lies in the median plane, which divides the head symmetrically, the impressions on either ear will be the same. All sounds in this plane ought therefore to produce a resultant of identical and indistinguishable transverse position, as they actually do. But the intensive height of this position (or at this position) and the gradient on either side of it will vary directly with the intensity and inversely with the distance of the sound from the head. Intensity and distance should therefore be indistinguishable in the median plane.

When the source lies elsewhere in the horizontal plane, the nearer ear will get the stronger impression. A leftward position will always produce a different effect from a rightward one. But for any left forward position there will always be a left rearward one (or a small region of them) that gives one and the same ratio of intensities and identical resultants. And similarly in the frontal plane for any left upward position of a sounding body a left downward one will always be found that yields the same resultant. The dependence of binaural position upon differences of intensity can readily be tested by placing a binaural stethoscope (or similar arrangement of tubes) upon a ticking watch and then pinching one of the tubes gradually. As the tube closes, the sound moves slowly round from the median plane in towards the unoccluded ear, until it seems to be

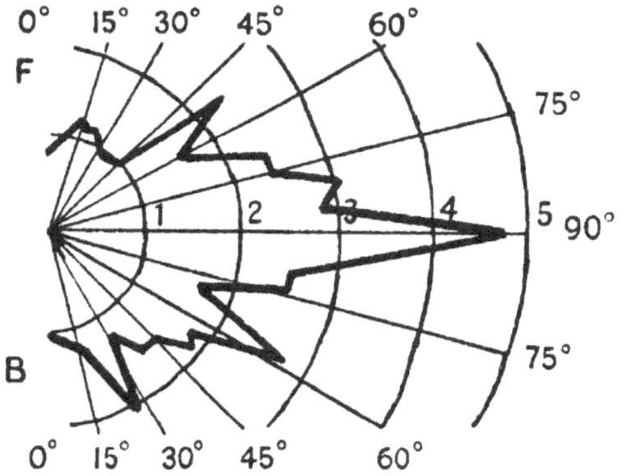

FIG. 15.—(From D. Starch, *Psych. Monog.*, 1905, 1 (4), p. 10. Cf. Seashore, *Elem. Experimts. in Psych.*, 1908, p. 60). The black line shows the number of degrees displacement (1, 2, 3, 4, 5) required for 75% right judgments as to displacement of the source of sound at a general distance of 1 metre from the head.

there altogether. The subject naturally is more impressed by the relative increase in the unchanged ear than by the decrease of intensity in the occluded ear. When the source of sound lies in the interaural axis both increase of intensity at the source and change of distance again produce only differences of resultant intensity, but not of binaural position. So here again these factors should tend to be confused with one another. These deductions are all readily verified by simple tests.

In daily life discrimination of binaural position seems, if anything, rather too fine for the differentiation of position by summation of unequal components that seems possible.

Fig. 15 shows how the threshold of discrimination rises and falls as we pass from straight in front, round by the right, to directly behind. It is lowest in front because it is easier to notice a slight departure from equality than to detect an increase in an already great difference (cf. Weber's law). So the threshold opposite either ear is high. If the head were a perfect sphere, the threshold would presumably rise and fall gradually between these extremes. The irregularities found are probably due to the square shape of the head and to the prominences of the external ear.

When the observer is prevented from knowing what sort of sound will next appear and where in the whole field it will probably lie, much less accuracy is shown in discriminating positions binaurally. Then, for example, seven

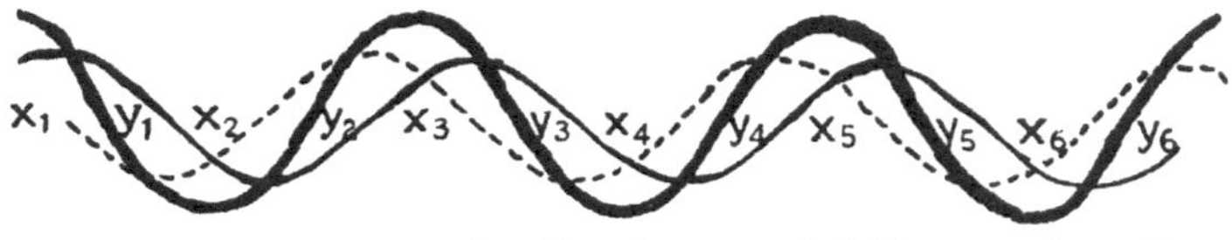

FIG. 16.—One ear leading by one-eighth wave-length. Thin line starts at R side. Dotted line starts at L side. Heavy line represents the standing wave that results from these two. From H. M. Halverson, *Psychol. Monog.* 1922, **31** (1) p. 8.

sounds are placed in front for one behind. And when a number of tones are sounded at once, only right and left are hardly ever misjudged. These irregular circumstances, however, undoubtedly coarsen our sense of binaural position. The native capacity of the ear will lie somewhere between these worst, and its best, performances.

Now for the dependence upon phase-differences. Suppose the interaural axis is lying on the line joining two telephone receivers emitting tones of the same pitch that differ from one another in phase by some fraction less than half a wave-length (cf. Fig. 16, where the fraction is one-eighth). A stationary wave is then formed on the line joining the two receivers; it is shown by the heavy black line in the figure. When the centre of the head (or the nose as indicator) lies at points such as X4 (" loops ") a phantom sound is heard that appears to lie high up (60°) in the median place, clear but remote. A slight shift of the head towards either Y3 or Y4 makes the phantom sound seem to move in a graceful curve in the same direction as the head. As Fig. 17 shows in the curved line, the phantom sweeps round towards the interaural axis, gradually changing in quality as it advances. From about 45° a second sound seems to reinforce it, growing in size and strength, until at 90° the phantom is quite enveloped and

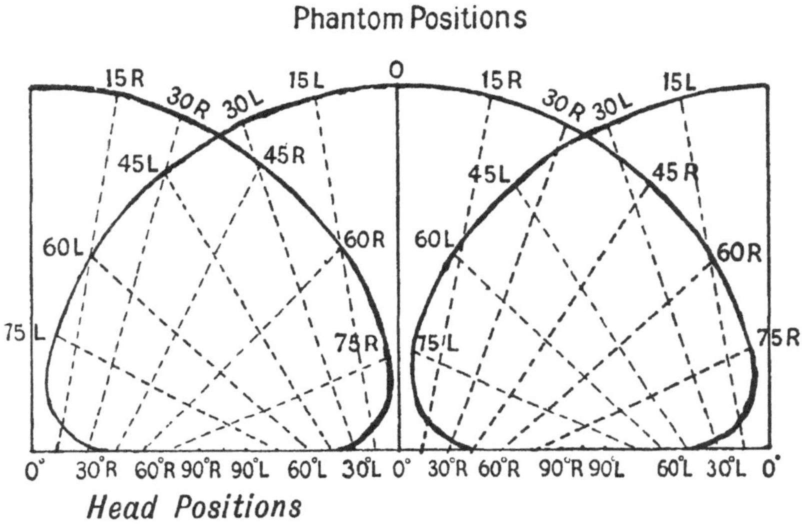

FIG. 17.—When the head moves from position O (on the base line) to position 15R, the phantom moves from the median plane to position 15R (on the curved line) relatively to the head. (Halverson, *ibid.*, p. 13.)

overwhelmed. Thereafter a third sound is heard at the left ear; this seems to grow in intensity until thereby the sound all seems to lie at the left ear. It is not so much a movement from ear to ear that takes place, as a rapid reduction of the one ear's sound in favour of the other. The sequence of changes from this point onwards is the exact reverse of that from the median plane to the right ear. The phantom first seems to emerge within the enveloping sound at about 75° left. And so on in cycles, as the figure shows. The quality, intensity, and extensity [1]

[1] Medianly localised tones, where the phase-difference is zero, and laterally localised tones, where the phase-difference is half the

of the tone at a node (at the ears) differs so much from the phantom at a loop (in the median plane) that for a practised observer there is no mistaking them. The cycle from median plane to median plane is completed in a movement of the head along half a wave-length between the receivers (from one X through a Y to the next X).

Variation of the intensity of tone emitted by the receivers produces a similar, though incomplete, series of changes, just as in the experiment with the watch and stethoscope. Now, however, the stimulus is tonal, not noisy. The quality of the tone changes greatly in the process. It begins as nearly pure and gradually becomes more and more complex until the entire sound occupies the right ear. It moves about 30° from the median position and reaches the aural axis when the difference of intensities has become great. The former movement is continuous, transition to the extreme position is discontinuous.

Whereas with ordinary means of stimulation through the air, noises give much clearer changes of binaural position than tones, with the method of phase changes the contrary holds. When a tone contains strong overtones, an extraordinary effect is produced. Each partial then moves about the head (as the latter is moved towards one of the receivers) at the rate set by its own wave-length. The first partial moves like the fundamental through a complete semicircle from one end of the interaural axis to the other. But the "image" of the second partial moves only over an arc of about 90° from 45° to the one side to 45° to the other.[1] And so there is a complex coming and going of these partial tones around the head, the octave partial moving at twice the rate of the fundamental and so on according to their relative rates of vibration.

wave-length, are of greatest volume and intensity. The intermediate phase-differences give smaller tones, the minimal volume occurring for a difference in phase of about $\frac{3}{16}$ wave-length. These volumic changes are of the same kind as the changes of volume that accompany changes of pitch. (H. M. Halverson, *Amer. J. Psych.*, 1922, **33**, 526 ff.) What the relation of these changes of volume is to those that accompany pitch, is not yet clear. They seem to be connected with our judgment of distance, and invite comparison with the analogous relations of apparent size and distance in vision.

[1] H. M. Halverson, *Amer. J. Psych.*, 1922, **33**, 178 ff.

Finally it is important to notice that the relative intensity effect and the relative phase effect on binaural position are neither completely continuous nor concomitant. The intensity effect does not exist for all frequencies from 200 to 4000 vbs. for all individuals. Ten out of sixteen observers found that the rotation of the apparent sound about the head ceased in a certain region or regions within this range. The bands of lapse vary in breadth and location in the range, but with one exception all occur above 800 vbs. There are frequency bands that give but one phantom, whose displacement from the median plane depends on the ratio of intensities at the ears. And there are others wherein two phantoms are formed, one stationary in the median plane and the other rotating as in the case of the single fusion.

But up to a frequency of some 1200 vbs. intensity seems to be a much less important factor in binaural position than phase. There is an upper frequency limit to the phase effect, averaging 1200 vbs. for sixteen observers. The effect does not seem to recur at higher frequencies. With six of the sixteen observers the phase effect continued through at least a portion of the lapse region for the intensity effect. These facts seem to exclude any explanation of phase effect in terms of intensity. "The organs of hearing must respond to phase as such, since phase and intensity are the only physical variations possible in a pure tone."[1]

This conclusion, however, is not quite compelling. It is possible that each of these factors may act upon the same mechanism of the ear and yet this mechanism may be differently accessible to the action of each. But we can hardly discuss this problem until we have some idea how phase differences reach the ear and the receptors of hearing. Until we have clearer ideas of the mechanism affected by phase differences, we cannot form any useful idea of the psychophysical processes involved. But we can be sure from the psychological side that, even if there be two physical factors, there is only one psychological resultant —viz. differences in binaural position. That alone enables us to affirm that the two factors must finally reach one and the same psychophysical mechanism.

[1] G. W. Stewart, *Psych. Monographs*, 1922, Vol. XXI, p. 44.

It is not yet clear whether the differentiation of positions given by intensity are equal to, or different from, those given by phase. One would surmise from the experimental records that the latter is finer. But, as no difference has yet been declared, it may well be that they are equally fine. This would support the theory of one psychophysical mechanism acted upon by two different physical variants.

If binaural position were dependent solely upon such differences of intensity as are given by a source of sound lying at different places about the head, it is clear that at all points between the median plane and the interaural axis there would be an intermingling of the effects of place in the horizontal plane and of distance from the head. For at great distances the impressions of either ear would become practically identical and so the sound would necessarily acquire a median position. But we know from daily experience that that does not happen. And it is obvious that phase differences would be entirely unaltered no matter how far away the source of sound were. How valuable this medium of differential stimulation must therefore be for binaural position ! Whether a pure distance factor in binaural hearing exists, is still uncertain. The observations of daily life would seem to suggest it, but whether it depends upon " experience " or not, we do not yet know.

Thus far we have been concerned with what we may call the direct and specific position of sounds. The sound, as determined by differences of intensity or phase, presents itself to us as of a certain position. We do not need to reflect or to infer its position from any peculiarities in the sound other than the position it actually occupies. But many considerations, both physical and psychological, impel us to look for another means of ascribing position to sounds or of localising them. This means is by contrast indirect : we ascribe a position to a sound, not by observing in it its position, but by inferring on the basis of memory or " experience " that sounds of that peculiar nature are such as we have by other means previously found to be located physically in such and such positions.

The basis of indirect localisation by inference is the changes in the blend of partials in sounds under varying circumstances. The head probably screens off or weakens some of the higher partials, just as a door or window does. Near sounds, like near colours, seem fuller and richer. Persons who have been trained to recognise the place in the median plane from which a sound comes—by their having the sound and the name of its place given to them many times over—declare that their estimates are based upon such subtle changes in blend. And the threshold of differentiation of position round the head for tones, especially pure tones, is very much higher (rougher) than for noises.

The theory of binaural position cannot be finally summed up in definite terms owing to the present fluid state of our knowledge. But both intensity and phase differences seem to give us nothing more than a line of positions (" transverse " to the musical dimension). Whether the circular movement in towards the head under phase changes is illusory, we can hardly say. But it is important that the phantom sound seems to lie out in front and it does not swing out to behind the head. By the aid of other senses and by our familiarity with the usual intensity of common sounds we learn to " project " these positions to a distance, whereby a sound seems to lie in a certain direction from us. Ambiguities still remaining are resolved by our experiences of the changes of blend that follow changes of position indicated through other channels than hearing. So we distinguish front from back, up and down on the same side, and other degrees of deviation horizontally about the head.

To help out the resolution of ambiguities that still remain various other signs have been invoked, as for example the touch sensations caused by sounds playing on the head, external ears and drums. But these do not seem to be prominent enough to be effective.

Another peculiar fact is the intracranial localisation that sounds often exhibit in experiments. It comes with force and surprise to those who, never having noticed it before, could hardly have learnt to infer it from anything else. It also points to some other direct factor, but not to a substitute for the direct factor ; for intracranial localisations show the same range of differences as extracranial ones. We need some " sign " merely for " in " rather than " out."

If we adopt the theory of binaural position by overlapping and summation, we may now conclude that *both* the dimensions of the auditory field provide differences of position. And from the point of view of the elementary attributes of sensation both dimensions are the same in nature in spite of their enormous differences of length. Longitudinal positions we know as pitches; they never become anything more than they are in themselves originally. Transverse positions are familiarly known as locations about the head, but they do not start as such. Primarily they are merely positions in the transverse aspect. But by entering into correlation with positions given in the other senses they become locations. In other words the further complications of experience bring them into different settings, and it is from these that they have received their characteristic names. These settings, however, as we shall see, do not alter or prevent their original being or essence. The elements that make up complex experiences do not seem to be altered or to disappear in the process in spite of the new experiences that appear with their integration or that their integration constitutes. Thus we find traces of a conservation of the elements of experience in their combinations in spite of the great changes and differences between them that these combinations seem to imply. Who would think that pitch and location of sounds are fundamentally the same thing? The sameness has indeed been felt " intuitively," as the use of the terms pitch, height, etc., imply. But even those who tried to read pitch as position had the greatest difficulty in persuading themselves to do so. We find this same sameness in the case of melody and motion and in other subtler cases that experiment reveals. We shall doubtless find it often again as psychology gradually succeeds in laying bare the architecture of mind.

Thus we understand better why only such sounds as differ in pitch can be properly localised when they occur simultaneously. For only these lie at different points of the length of the auditory field and so stand free of one another. Identical sounds sum their forces in either ear and give rise to a single phantom sound that is placed according to the final resultant of all the partial intensities. And the volumes of tones are not heard as lengths of space at the place where the sound is heard to lie. For the functions of the longitudinal and the transverse aspects of the auditory field are so different, the one being musical, the other positional or spatial, that they are kept apart in our minds, as we shall consider more fully later on.

CHAPTER XIII

THE THIRD DIMENSION OF VISUAL POSITION

IT is easy to prove that a single stationary eye over against a field of motionless objects presents us with only two dimensions of visual position. Hang a number of small spheres (e.g. walnuts) of different sizes from invisible threads before a plain background, and set the spheres irregularly with reference to their size and their distance from the eye. Uniocular vision will then fail to reveal the relative positions of the spheres in the line of sight. The same fact may be noticed on looking with one eye into a leafy bush ; it seems as "flat" as it would in a photograph. But when we look at these things with both eyes at once, the relative positions of each part in the line of sight stand out very clearly indeed. We actually see another—a third—dimension of positions or distances.

Now this third dimension is obviously an addition to the differences of position that under the circumstances either eye alone can provide. It also unifies the data obtained by the two eyes and it is referred or attached to them. So it conforms to the features of the process of integration that we distinguished above (p. 75). To these we may now add a third feature, which we suggest provisionally as characteristic of integration : the new feature resembles the data it unifies and integrates ; it seems to be almost an extension of them in a new direction. If we go on to note that the process of integration is spontaneous, we do not thereby establish any further positive characteristic of it. We merely assert that the third dimension of position is not brought about by any force or process that is external to the data which integrate, whether this be some power of attention or some process or activity of the "mind" or of the self, or the like. Even if such powers, distinguishable from the integrating data themselves, seem able at times to support or to oppose the process of integration, we certainly cannot hope to prove that they initiate it and sustain it entirely. Any such thesis would be inconsistent with the natural logic of explanation, which is essentially positivistic and economical.

As in the study of binaural position so here we have to distinguish actual positions from signs of position. Such signs are provided by differences of visual size, by perspective, by differences of saturation and brightness, by shadows and overlapping contours. Distant objects look smaller, and all lines that are parallel to the level line of sight converge on a point on the horizon—the vanishing point, constituting the system of relations known as perspective. Between the eye and any surface float innumerable specks of matter that all reflect some light. The further away an object is, therefore, the more white light will be mixed with the light it reflects and the less saturated will its colour appear. Thus decrease of saturation is a sign of distance. But we have to learn all these signs, whereas there is nothing to learn about the third dimension of visual positions. It is simply given to us.

We must now consider how the two eyes work together to establish this process of stereoscopic integration. In the two ears the task was simpler. For they are fixed structures, as passively subject to the action of physical sound as the skin is to any degree of warmth of the surrounding air. But the eyes are extremely mobile organs, delicately balanced upon their muscles and in constant movement under their changes of innervation. And yet their movements are so well co-ordinated that they seem to act like one thing. How is this co-ordination attained ? It does not begin at birth ; it has apparently to be learnt by the infant ; and it can be altered when it is upset by the defects that end in squinting.

The primary condition of co-ordination is undoubtedly the distribution of sensitivity over the retina. Acuity of vision is greatest at the fovea centralis. From there outwards in all directions it diminishes rapidly. If you steadily fixate some point on a line of print, you can see clearly only a letter or two on either side of it. Further out you can see only the forms of the words as a whole, though you can still read some of them quite confidently. You can only guess at the remoter ones. The same holds rather less for the letters and words above and below the point of fixation.

Now the eyes constantly readjust themselves in the act of vision so that the object of attention falls partly or wholly within the clearest area. The object of attention is primarily the object that most compels action, especially the brightest stimulus. Upon this basis determining processes are built up that in the adult mind become the apparently free work of attention. When the attention passes to another point, the eyes move together so as to bring it on to the fovea. One or more very small corrective movements may follow the first large adjustment. Even when one eye is occluded, it is automatically set and adjusted for the object at which the other eye is looking, as the familar test for heterophoria implies. One eye is covered with the hand while the other eye sees the flame of a candle through the Maddox multiple rod as a long vertical streak. When the hand is quickly removed, the streak will be seen to run vertically through the middle of the candle flame, if the co-ordination of the eyes is normal. If not, the streak will lie some distance to the right or left of the flame, according as the free eye converges or diverges a little from the normal line of sight. Very often upon exposure it quickly moves into the correct posture.

The co-ordination of the eyes is therefore normally very good. But it does not seem to be perfect. Photographic registration and measurement of the movements of the eyes show that even when they are fixating a point steadily and clearly, and seeing it sharply and singly, they may change their convergence very slightly. Or in the changing of fixation the one eye may move a little ahead of the other. These are, of course, degrees of heterophoria ; but they seem to be normal degrees. If they did not exist, we should have to infer that the two eyes were co-ordinated with mathematical precision with one another, so that with one point (or cone) on the one retina only one single point on the other would give single vision for any fixed distance.

That does not seem to be true. A small area of points corresponds to any one point in the other eye.

As a rough general rule single vision results from the stimulation of points on either retina that lie equally far in the same direction from their respective foveas. The discrepancy is rather marked only in the vertical dimension. This rule is known as the correspondence of the retinas. Its equivalent in the field of vision is the horopter, all points in which appear single to both eyes if one of them does.

As the eyes stand at a certain distance from each other in the head, they get different views of the objects observed. One eye sees more of the right aspect, the other of the left. Suppose the eyes to be looking at a pyramid having its apex towards them, then the right eye will see the rightward surface of the four that meet in an apex broader than the leftward one; the left eye contrariwise (Fig. 18).

FIG. 18.

These two views differ laterally, i.e. in a line parallel to that occupied by the two eyes. If one of two points lies nearer the head than another, one of the eyes will see these points as if they were closer together than the other will. The rule of this disparity of images is very simple: if a distance is greater in the left (right) field of vision, the left (right) bounding point will be farther away from us. If it is smaller, the latter point will be nearer. This may be verified in Fig. 18. The rule holds when one of the distances dwindles to nothing (to a mere point) or even when it becomes negative, i.e. when the left point for one eye is for the other eye the right point (i.e. when the two points lie one behind the other in the median plane). But these cases are apt to fall to pieces on examination; they need the help of fluent action in stereoscopic observation.

Such special cases accentuate a problem of fundamental importance for theory. By what sign do the eyes know—

to express it crudely—which point in the one field of vision belongs to which in the other? We can easily isolate the primary sign if we make a stereogram for a swarm of points at different distances from the observer. Then it can only be the disposition of the points in the two fields, i.e. the equality or slight disparity of their *distances* from one another in the same direction in either field. Hereby each point finds its partner in the other field independently of all the rest of the points, on the basis of mere proximity of distance. But points in either field can be linked together by intervening points or by lines in such a way that this rule of proximity seems to be overruled. Of course, it is not really overruled; for the closely neighbouring points, or the continuous series of the points of a line determine changes of fixation and thereby the resulting stereoscopy. The latter, however, is always governed by the limits of the disparity compatible with single stereoscopic vision.

These limits may be noticed when we gaze with both eyes steadily at the apex of a real pyramid or of a pyramid in a stereogram (cf. Fig. 18). The lines radiating from it appear double further along, gradually diverging from the apex. If we move our vision along these lines, we see that the single point moves with us, the lines beginning to cross and then finally converging at the corner of the base in the directions opposed to their previous divergence. The apex now is double and the base corner and lines single. But the pyramid looks solid all the time. It seems single and solid for some distance on either side of (nearer and farther than) the point fixated, and double at greater distances. This single and solid region (which extends from the fovea into the periphery of the field of vision about 10°) we may call the solid or stereoscopic zone. As the point of fixation moves gradually or leaps (as it does habitually), this zone slides to and fro or leaps, making single what was previously double.

But ordinarily we do not notice the doubling at all; in fact, we are usually unaware of its existence and have to make some effort to detect it. For our active interest is always in what is for the moment combinedly single. If our interest is attracted by what is at the moment double, our eyes move together to their new points of interest by a swift leap, during which no noticeable change of visual sensations supervenes. And these points then appear single. Wherever we look we see single objects. To see the double images that constantly form the greater part of our vision, we must make the unusual effort of divorcing our interests and our eye movements from conjoint action so as to change the former while maintaining one and the same fixation.

But why do we see single with two eyes at all? In hearing we did not need to state this question explicitly; for the answer to it is obviously implied in the theory of the psychophysical overlapping and summation of processes that we there adopted. When a pencil is pushed in between two closed fingers, we feel it as one, because the areas stimulated are next neighbours: each constitutes its mass of touch sensation and the two together form one whole that is for us the form of the pencil. When a pencil is inserted between crossed fingers, as in Aristotle's illusion, we feel it distinctly as two, because then the wood stimulates two areas that are normally distant from one another. But the eyes do not bring their fields into any overlapping and summation, even though the combined field of vision is functionally binocular in the middle and uniocular on either side of that, just like the binaural field. Nor are the two eyes next neighbouring parts of one larger field although the three parts of the combined field of vision—uniocular, binocular, uniocular, are such next neighbours. Under ordinary circumstances the intensity of the binocular field is exactly the same as that of either field alone (if the sight of the latter is normal). It is for this reason that, as in Sherrington's experiments, the brightness that results from the fusion of dark and light phases that are binocularly alternate is the same as results when they are binocularly synchronous, and the rate of succession required for the fusion is the same in both cases. Binocular vision, however, is rather better than uniocular, in so far as we ordinarily take from each field what is best in it: i.e. it is finer and clearer, not brighter or lighter. We must therefore look for some other basis of psychophysical unity than the rather mechanical ones we have met with already.

Vision is peculiar in that one eye may be diverted from its usual co-ordination by the push of a finger, when the previously single appears double, as if there were really two things side by side in space. When one eye is too large for its socket or its muscles are too weak or its vision very bad, co-ordination is either never completed by the individual's effort of learning in infancy, or what was gained is lost, and squinting with its double images supervenes. The subject may learn to overcome the confusion thus produced by ignoring one of the two images. H' will generally attend to the one that is clearer, i.e. the one that is centred on the fovea of its eye. His vision then may become alternate, just as it is in normal eyes if we look now to the extreme right now to the extreme left, without moving the head, or if we attend to these quarters without moving the eyes at all. In normal eyes the vision of both eyes persists all the time, of course. But in some squinters the bad eye is for the moment so neglected that it might almost as well be blind. And yet careful tests (e.g. the ordinary tests for rivalry of images—a black horizontal line shown to one eye and a vertical one to the other) will show that both eyes can still see at once. In other cases of squinting one of the two eyes does become functionally blind. If the tendency towards this complete neglect of one eye is detected in time, the dwindling remnant of interest in its vision can be restored by practice. For this purpose the good eye is covered for a few minutes at a time while the other eye is made to follow a light, etc. Thus the child learns again to direct this eye's clearest part upon the object of interest and so to co-ordinate the movements of the eyes in spite of any little obstruction or weakness in one of them.

In a third group of cases a new correspondence is established between the fields of vision. The fovea of the good eye now sees single in co-operation with a point in the bad eye that lies some distance away from its fovea (according to the size of the angle of squint). And all the points of the bad eye correspond with points in the good eye accordingly. Obviously this adjustment is very much more difficult to attain, because it has to be won in spite of the distribution of clearness in the two fields. What the one eye sees clearly the other will see in a degree of unclearness that corresponds to the angle of squint. And so the lateral differences that ordinarily yield stereoscopy are practically never utilised properly again. The squinter lacks stereoscopic vision.

In hearing no such process of squinting is known. One ear may be put out of tune by catarrh of the middle ear, or the like. The same tune is then heard double in two pitches. But this effect—apart from certain necessary differences—is essentially the same as that produced by hearing (receiving) in either ear the same tune at these different pitches. The same may be said in analogous terms for the objects seen double in squinting vision or when a prism is set before either eye. But the peculiarity of vision is that the eye can be rotated and thus alone produce the doubleness. And the mistuning produced in hearing never disappears by the formation of a new correspondence. The overlapping and summation of hearing make that impossible.

In cases of hemianopsia Fuchs[1] found that a new fovea or pseudo-fovea was formed, from which clearness of vision decreased in all directions, including that towards the anatomical fovea. A small object shown a little towards the periphery appears blurred and unclear or is not seen at all. It grows clear or even visible only when it is taken up into a larger figure as a constituent part of it. Its clearness comes and goes with this figure. And the larger the object shown appears to be (not as a retinal image), the further outwards the pseudo-fovea moves.

[1] W. Fuchs, *Ztsch. Psych.*, 1919, **84**, 67 ff.; 1921, **86**, 1 ff.; *Psych. Forsch.*, 1921, **1**, 157 ff.

CHAPTER XIV

STEREOSCOPIC VISION

FROM these various facts and reflexions we may infer that it is the similarity of the visual forms in the two eyes and their similar changes from moment to moment that is the basis of single vision with two eyes. Any mechanical linkage of the two fields point for point together would make the squinter's change of correspondence impossible. If he has to achieve this change by way of the similarity of forms appearing in the two fields, we may infer that the child's unity of vision is established by the same means. Only the child is greatly aided by the grading of clearness from the fovea outwards, which is a compelling motive to co-ordination. That the squinter often reaches a new correspondence in spite of this irremovable circumstance shows how powerful a force for unification the identity of forms must be. So we must conclude that the two fields of vision are psychophysically identified, not summated or juxtaposed. It is a familiar fact of physiology that the fibres of the optic nerve cross over at the chiasma so that all points on the two retinas that lie to the left of a common central region are connected with the left hemisphere of the brain and all those that lie to the right with the right hemisphere. But we may not interpret this as if the fibres finally impinged upon the same cells of the cortex and there coalesced ; for that would imply the summation of the intensities of the two fields in binocular vision, which we know does not happen.

Indeed the identification of fields is a by-product of binocular vision that by itself would be superfluous. The essential function of binocular vision is stereoscopy, in which the differences of the two fields within certain limits are integrated and so yield a valuable addition to sensory experience. As we found in dealing with the first integrations of distance, it is extremely difficult to rationalise this process in integration. We cannot readily see what makes it come about or what is the inner spontaneity that resides in its contributory parts to make them assume solidity. In fact, it may well be impossible to render such spontaneity in conceptual terms. For it is individual and unique, one of a class of integrative processes no doubt, but an individual in that class. We can therefore only hope to state the features that are common to all integrative processes, not to seize the individuality of each completely. As was observed in the introduction to this book it is the fact, and the supreme importance, of integration in the scheme of mind that make so great a difference between the work of the psychologist and that of the physicist. The latter can follow his elements and their quantitative properties into all the complications they assume. And every known feature of the latter can be expressed in terms of the former. For no complication in the physical world appears to give rise to any really new property or substance. Units of complexity have therefore no quality in physics : their relations are all reducible to quantitative terms of the component elements, whatever they are. But in the world of mind every integration involves not only unification, but an addition to the stuff or substance of experience. Quantitative continuity can therefore never be finally attained, but only approximate continuity or identity of psychical stuff and properties from elements to complexities. The point of view of the pure psychologist is like that of the artist, not like that of the dynamical mechanist. He is most keenly interested in the " star " that is born of three things combined : the beauty, the value, the truth, the solidity that a grouping of experiences brings forth. Unlike the artist's, however, his interest does not end with the creative act ; it continues forth until all the conditions surrounding it have been exhaustively tested and tabulated according to the methods common to all science.

It is the difficulty naturally inherent in the study of integration that has impelled so many thinkers to try to explain stereoscopy and other integrations of all kinds externally, as it were. We feel we must look for some agent to work the process for us, it may be the linkage of neural processes in the brain, or the mysterious soul, or the intellect that on the basis of "experience" learns to connect the disparate group of images with the idea of solidity drawn from some other sense, such as the motor combination. But we know nothing as yet about these brain processes and could only infer them from our experiences of solidity. In any case we must first solve the psychological problems of stereoscopy before we can hope to undertake the physiological ones. Appeal to the soul or "subject" only passes the difficulty into the depths of obscurity. The ego seems a satisfying force to many thinkers, to be sure. For we feel that "we" are behind all our own mental processes, doing them and shaping them, moulding irregular and refractory material into intellectual and moral shape. Of course; but at the same time we all recognise that we do not make our own thoughts: they come to us, and we are active in their coming. We must speak of them all as "ours" if we are to maintain a distinction between them and those of other people whose thoughts we learn. Besides, who will explain to us how the "subject" could put two experiences together that were not of themselves natural complements, fit for integration? Where would the subject get the new feature, the integrate? And how would he implant it upon the integrating data? Surely it is easier and more logical to treat integration descriptively and inferentially, than it is to make such arbitrary assumptions that involve more mysteries than they explain.

In short, we cannot draw visual solidity (or any other integrative produce) from outside itself. It is native or autonomous, as all the fundamental processes of mind are. Explanation by heteronomy is the prevailing fashion of present psychology. And if the fact to be explained will not be drawn from some foreign source, the last resort is to treat it as illusory. Many attempts have been made to do this for stereoscopy, to show that it is only a more vivid form of the distance we get in any flat art (picture, etching, etc.), and really the product of attention and its processes, or associative reminiscences, and the like. But they all signally fail to explain away the fact of stereoscopic solidity, the fact that then one point is psychically really nearer than another and does not merely seem to be nearer while obviously at the same place (on the canvas, etc.), as in a picture.

It is more difficult in stereoscopy to trace the contributory parts than in simple distances, time-intervals, motions, or binaural positions. Double images point clearly towards them. Although some writers suppose that these images are not simultaneously, but only alternately, present, that is really a mistake, as observation shows. Of course if we gaze at them too staringly, they will alternate. But they do not do so readily.

Perhaps from the rule governing the disparity of the two fields we can come closest to a theory of the inner nature of stereoscopy. " If a distance is greater in the left (right) field of vision, the left (right) bounding point of it will be farther away." This increase of size appears in the integration of the distances as a new kind of size, a variant of the kind of size whose differences are integrated.

Vertical disparity, though it is easy to arrange experimentally, does not yield stereoscopic vision. For it is a perfectly ambiguous arrangement. The rule would now read : if the distance in the left field is greater, the upper point will be farther away. But why farther and not nearer. There is nothing left " to guide our choice " ; whereas, in spite of the mystery of integration in general, the rule of lateral disparity does seem more rational in that left and left, right and right go together in it. The rational, however, cannot be a final test in such matters. For stereoscopy is not a process of reason. These (of reason) are distinct and unique processes of mind. And we can no more take reason as a final measure of stereoscopy than we can set up red as the measure of blue or blue of sweet. This is, of course, the " reason " for the fallacy of rationalism generally. Nevertheless in so far as reason seeks for conditioning differences, it is on sound lines. For these differences are common to all events. Reason is then merely doing its own work, not trying to turn itself into something other than itself.

Perhaps we might feel inclined to claim merely that the

peculiar increase of size enfolded in the integration of distances from either eye is primarily merely an unknown meaningless variant, which afterwards comes to " mean " farther away, because it enters into all those connexions that constitute space and its sensory relations (cf. Chap. XVIII). But this would again imply surrender to the illusion of explaining a feature of vision from without. And it would not help us the more to penetrate the mystery of the added feature in integration. In final desperation we may appeal to physiological speculation and assume that disparate points take up positions in the cortex that in the real substance of it lie in the third dimension relatively to the two plane dimensions of either eye. Thus stereoscopy would have the same sort of physiological basis as any plane distance presumably has. Presumably! But what is the physiological presumption for even the plane distances? Not just being a distance between excitations, surely! If not, then we are as far from finally understanding the process physiologically as psychologically. The solid physiological basis is too easy an explanation even if it were in the least probable.

The two halves of the stereogram of any *geometrical* figure can be interchanged without any loss of stereoscopic effect. Of course the whole system of stereoscopic relations is thereby reversed. But with the stereogram of a landscape the reversal is not nearly so good. It occurs quite definitely in various parts of the picture, especially in the foreground where disparity is greatest. But it is never properly systematic as it is in geometrical forms or in stereograms of the moon and such unperspectival objects. With practice and persistence the stereoscopy of the reversed landscape increases greatly. But it is difficult, for it involves a conflict between acts of observation, especially eye-movements, and trains of interpretative acts or impulses. We cannot well prepare our perception to look for perspectivally small objects in the foreground or for trees and men directly behind walls or houses or for a ground that slopes from high-up to low-down and that forms a screen of atmosphere through which all objects are to be seen, and so on.

It is therefore evident that stereoscopic effects may be produced in different degrees by the mutual co-operation or opposition of such factors as can suggest depth strongly, and serve to guide our observation of it in an orderly way, like that which we have learnt by the long practice of life, or that on the contrary suggest flat surfaces and confuse our orderly observation. A single figure that we know only as a flat object will not "suggest" depth; but one that represents a possible solid object, or either of two opposite (reversed) solids, will give a stronger idea of depth; and a photograph or picture of a courtyard or landscape, etc., will do this more easily. But no part of the landscape appears to lie in front of the canvas or behind it. Nor does this happen in the figure of cubes (Fig. 9, p. 83); it is still all on the surface of the paper, though variously solid in appearance. It is only when we turn to figures involving two disparate images, e.g. the familiar "plastographic album" in which the left and right eye views are printed in red and green above one another, the stereoscope in its various forms, and natural perception of space, that one figure actually is nearer in the field of vision than another. And any form of the stereoscope that gets rid in increasing degrees of the flattening effect of the paper of the prints and the marks on it and that introduces the adjuvant factors of familiar figures and all the secondary suggestions of depth (colour saturation, brightness, shadows, etc.) will give an increasingly vivid depth. But depth does not grow gradually out of flatness by each factor adding its own little bit of depth to the whole. Retinal disparity is the essential requisite for the emergence of real psychical depth.

In the stereoscope we still see the plane of the paper cutting the solid figure in two with a more or less distinct surface. And the sides of the figure sometimes seem to possess a sort of transparent surface. This is similar to the surface of glass [1] seen when we look through a window at a landscape, especially in moving the head laterally, or to the surface that may be seen even in a fine mirror when we attend to its surface rather than to what we see in it. In the paper of the stereogram, the window, the mirror, these surfaces are optically presented, of course. In the pro-

[1] Cf. Schumann, *Ztsch.*, 1920, **85**, 224 ff.

truding or receding surfaces of the stereoscopic solid they have to be borrowed from the optical presentations. But they cannot constitute the basis of " empty space," i.e. of solidity or third dimension as such. For they only become planes in a solid by the prior " creation " of solidity, which concretes them out of what is optically presented in two dimensions.

A curious relation between stereoscopy and visual brightness occurs. When a rod is moved in front of a bright background on a line perpendicular to the line of sight, it appears to move in a straight line only when it is equally bright for both eyes. Otherwise it seems to move in a circle, for the darker stimulus is later in arousing its sensation and so creates a lateral disparity. A delicate method of photometry is based upon this fact.[1]

Since there are physiological limits to our discrimination of differences of distance, the physical range of stereoscopic vision is limited by the distance between the eyes. It can be increased by virtual change in this distance, as in the range-finder. Normally it extends to about two kilometres, but the nearer point must then be about half that distance nearer. For this test all secondary indications of depth—perspective, changes of colour and brightness, shadows, overlapping of contours must be eliminated, and all view of the ground must be cut off by making the observer look over the edge of a card or wall at the two spheres or stakes.

When the eye or the objects of vision are moved against one another, as when a bird flies through the air, the same differences that appear simultaneously (and discretely) in binocular stereoscopy, are presented successively and *progressively*. A cinema that has been moved continuously across or past the scenes it has photographed, presents a series of this kind. And we notice in its display an excellent stereoscopic presentation even if we look at it with only one eye. We may therefore infer that the bird has a stereoscopic view of the things around it, even though it sees very few things with both eyes at once, especially when its eyes look out almost directly towards opposite sides. Our eyes lie as far apart as possible on the same side of the head so

[1] C. Pulfrich, as reported *Psych. Bull.*, 1922, **19**, 369 f.

that a large part of our total field of vision is binocular and stereoscopic. The rest merely extends this binocular part as if the whole field of vision belonged to one retina made up of neighbouring parts ; and these uniocular parts will be stereoscopic only under proper conditions of motion. In the eyes of many birds, fishes, etc., a much smaller part, different in size for different species, is binocular. The uniocular parts capable of producing " progressive " stereoscopy only, are much larger. The ideal or extreme eye of this type would be one that gets a complete panorama, spherical to the head. Animals with this type of vision must clearly be such as have more need of stereoscopic vision while they are in motion than while they are at rest. We belong to the converse class whose stereoscopic vision may be described as " static," along with all creatures that must estimate distances while they are still at rest.

In progressive stereoscopy similarity of distances or of forms plays even a more important part than in the static binocular process. If a complex of mere points is presented progressively to one eye, the optical result is hardly distinguishable from a flat group of points in irregular motion. There is nothing to distinguish between irregular motion of the points amongst one another and that systematic alteration of apparent position that is due to the eye and the group of objects moving over against one another. And of course it would be more difficult still to distinguish between the latter change as it would affect a group of objects in motion relatively to one another and such relative motion. Yet if it is to be of use progressive stereoscopy must be able to differentiate these two motions. This is possible only with the filled-out line- and mass-forms of geometrical figures or still more of everyday vision. Then what seemed to belie the systematic nature of binocular stereoscopic vision by refusing to be reversed by interchange of the images of either eye, for a similar reason helps to bind the points of successive uniocular forms firmly together and so distinguishes motions in any frontal plane clearly in the integrate from any motions in the stereoscopic plane.

The difference between static and progressive stereoscopy is simply the reappearance, on the higher level of integration, of the difference between distances that are based upon points presented simultaneously and those that involve successive presentation. So long as the rate of succession of the integrating sensations in these cases is not too slow, the succession produces no disturbing effect upon their integration. If it is too slow, the sensations are no longer together and so do not fulfil the first condition of integration. Otherwise in such integrations as these that are based ultimately upon differences of systemic position, time is simply irrelevant, because it does not form an essential ingredient of them.

Although we are right in saying that stereoscopy is based ultimately upon differences of systemic position, it actually consists of the integration of systemic *distances* as such or as implicit in lines, masses and plane forms. For that reason we are justified in viewing it as a higher level of integration than that in which distance itself first appears as integrate.

Only one other sense seems to be capable of providing figures in three as well as in two dimensions, namely, articular sense. The various limbs and joints of the body undoubtedly give together a complex figure of positions in three dimensions. That we can easily test by bringing a finger of one hand to meet a finger of the other at points behind, above, and below us that are not ordinarily or at the moment visible. They meet with considerable accuracy. One joint must, therefore, act as an extension or refinement of the previous. The hip, for instance, gives us about three quadrants of a circle of positions when it is swung in a circle about the other leg. When it is stopped in any position and the knee is then moved, the latter gives us a line of positions at that point of arrest. As articular sense is ultimately based upon sensations of skin pressure, the complexes of changes that constitute the positions of a joint lie embedded in the systemic field of touch and are used to characterise and modify the parts of it that are involved in the parts moving in each joint. The flexion or extension of a limb causes tensions and compressions on either side of the joint at varying distances from it, and in varying extents that we cannot yet describe accurately. But they seem to be sufficiently constant for the different degrees of flexion to act as a clear and delicate indication of posture and movement. No one joint, of course, gives three dimensions of variation, but only two at the most, in many cases only one. But three directions are readily established by the continuity of tension into neighbouring joint areas over the two dimensional field of pressure sense, so that articular sense functions easily and independently as a tridimensional sense. Delicacy of pressure sensitivity and freedom of movement are no doubt necessary conditions for the establishment of it as such.

CHAPTER XV

SINGLE SENSE INTEGRATIONS IN GENERAL

WE have now studied all the complexities that appertain to the senses singly or with the help of the doubling of complex organs like the ear and the eye. We may therefore now make a second table of the complexities of sense to show their order of complication, and their connexion with the attributes of the elements of sensation.

The two attributes of quality and intensity have been omitted from the table because they show little sign of progressive integration.

The case of lustre is of peculiar interest in this connexion. It makes some claim to be an integration of the qualities of vision. It is a peculiar combination of colours of different brightness, e.g. white and black, white and blue, light yellow and dark yellow. It can readily be obtained by presenting black and white surfaces to either eye in the stereoscope, if these are supported by some stereoscopic combination, as when the surfaces of a solid figure are set out in black and white alternately for either eye. Without the help of stereoscopy these black and white surfaces show the phenomena of visual rivalry: the black of the one eye occupies the field of vision alone for a time, while the white from the other eye is almost entirely suppressed; then the white gradually emerges while the black recedes completely for a time, and so on alternately with various local mixtures and wave-like changes. This rivalry is found in all binocular presentations that fail to procure stereoscopy at all. But rivalry is probably not, as some think, a fundamental process of vision that characterises even the stablest stereoscopy. In the latter, steady presence and union of both contributory presentations is

TABLE 3. SINGLE-SENSE INTEGRATIONS

Attributes of the elements	Minimal particles of	Systemic position-extent	Integration of systemic and temporal	Temporal position-extent
	Minimal aggregation.	Lines of one dimensional, or masses of two dimensional, more or less definite *size*.[1]	Motions of more or less definite *speed*.	Durations of more or less definite *size*.
1st level of integration endosystemic (single sense).	Manifold aggregation.	Lines or masses (areas, volumes) of definite *size*, outline, form.	Continuous motions of definite *speed*.	Durations of definite *size*.
	Clear distinction.	Distances, forms, figures.	If the separations are not too great, still continuous motions of reduced intensity. Otherwise more or less interrupted motions in systemic and temporal forms, e.g. melodies.	Intervals. Rhythms.
	Interaction of units(?)	Illusions of size, e.g. "filled and empty distance," Muller-Lyer, etc.	Illusions of speed (?) "of interrupted and continuous motions." (?)	Illusions of size, e.g. "filled and empty time."
Disystemic (two systems of the same sense, e.g. in vision.	Integration of products of first level.	Stereoscopy a third dimension of positions.	Nothing more, because of lack of further temporal development. But, of course, motions of the one and only kind ("simple") in the third dimension, e.g. in stereoscopy, will occur.	There is no further development.
		Etcetera.		

[1] Binaural position falls between this grade and the one below, rather nearer the former.

to be presumed, since the alterations in rivalry are very much slower than the longest alternate lapses (three or four a second) of either field of vision that may be caused without detriment to binocular stereoscopy (e.g. by rotating a suitably cut disc before the eyes). Besides no rivalry is to be observed in binocular stereoscopic vision until the conditions approach those of rivalry by difference of presentations.

Lustre seems in fact to confirm the view that in binocular vision the contributions of both fields of vision are normally present as actual sensations. For it is best described as the simultaneous presence of black and white in two different sheets at the same place in the binocular field.[1] The sheets may be continuously black and white or each sheet (as in the ordinary lustre of metallic surfaces) may be finely mottled black and white, the specks of the light in the one sheet being dark in the other sheet and vice versa. So lustre differs from grey, that looks like, and probably is, the simultaneous presence in a single sheet of minute black and white specks, that are presumably much finer than the specks of natural lustre. And when the two eyes look at a grey surface each sees the same kind of sheet in which there is no possibility of any distinctive presence in the one sheet of a white speck, where in the other there is a black one.

Lustre can also be produced uniocularly, if there is an alternation of light and dark phases at the same place in the visual field. This effect is produced when we look at the surface of running or rippling water and similar objects. It can be imitated with larger areas of black and white presented alternately, e.g. in a circular band in the middle of a rotating disc. A slow rate of alternation, some three or four times a second, gives quite a good uniocular lustre. If the rate is slower, we simply see black and white alternately. Metallic surfaces fixated steadily by a single eye look lustrous when they seem to the observer to reflect light from points not on their surfaces.[2] Metallic lustre is then a product of the perceptual analysis of the total light physically reflected by the object, which analysis

[1] S. Dawson, *Br. J. Psych.*, 1917, **8**, 510 ff.; 1918, **9**, 1 ff.
[2] Kirschmann, *Arch. ges. Psych.*, 1921, **41**, 90 ff.

is primarily constituted by the different brightness presented by such reflecting surfaces to binocular vision or in succession to uniocular vision. The stereoscope is unable to imitate metallic lustre.

Lustre, then, is not so much a new quality of vision as a special binding together of (brightness) differences in (uniocular) successive or (binocular) simultaneous sensations. The binding is not due to any will or desire or voluntary attention on our part, or to the "mind" in this sense of the term. Nevertheless it does not deserve the title of integration, any more than does the binaural series of positions. For, as in the latter, the end result is probably no more than the mere sum of the contributory parts, whereas in an integration (like stereoscopy) something distinctively new accrues upon the union of the contributory parts. Lustre certainly gives a new "effect," just as binaural hearing does, but it seems after all to be merely a special kind of sum-total of its constituents. The same conclusion probably applies to the combination of skin qualities, warmth and cold, that constitutes heat.

It is evident that the problem of lustre as an integration is independent of the question whether brightness in vision should be classified as a variant of quality or of intensity. We have seen that its closest affinity is probably to quality (cf. above, p. 56). There seems to be no other possible case of intensive integration. But there are several of quality. There is no à priori reason why intensity or quality should not integrate. The question is one of fact only, sifted and tested, of course, by analysis, classification, and systematic coherence.

It has been suggested that the "taste" of lemonade that contains sweet, sour, and a certain smell, is not these three sensations in a bunch, "but a star," a unique combination with a special character of its own. We may safely doubt this. Repeated trial with heat offers no obvious reason [1] for believing that heat contains some new feature beyond the warmth and cold that are undoubtedly there, no matter how strange it has been to discover that

[1] But the minute observations recently recorded by Cutolo would contradict this. Cf. above, p. 28.

heat does contain cold. What we learn to recognise and to name practically is the group as a characteristic whole.[1] Difficult combinations are also found in great numbers in the flavours of daily life. Taste and smell are commonly said to fuse together almost indistinguishably (apart from experiments by exclusion). But the difficulty is not to say whether lemonade is sweet or lemony, but to say whether lemonade smells sweet or only tastes sweet, tastes lemony or only smells so; i.e. to say which component is due to the tongue organs and which to those of the nasal cavity. We generally treat tastes and smells as if they belonged all to one "sense" as do the colours. Besides the difficulty is more real than it has often seemed to be. For it has been shown that in the nasal cavity there are actually taste organs that can be stimulated (during complete exclusion of the usual organs on the tongue) by much smaller quantities of substance and in a gaseous state. So we really do smell (or sniff) things sweet, sour and bitter, and things taste spicy, burnt, fruity, etc., although there is no regio olfactoria in the mouth. Of course the closest fusion between taste and smell occurs when both are nasal. Only, in these cases, as in the fusion of tones, we have to do with a mere sum, a combination in which the constituents are readily found and nothing beyond them. The same applies to the various forms of synæsthesia that have been described, e.g. coloured hearing or coloured taste, when sounds or tastes arouse the idea, sometimes almost the sensation, of some colour that changes with change of pitch or taste, etc. These probably rest upon chance associations formed in early youth, whose origins have been forgotten.

Closely allied to the problems of lustre is the study of binocular colour mixture. The mixture of neighbouring colours, such as red and orange, or blue and violet, does not produce any new style of colour, but merely the intermediate one that would result from the mixture of the same colours in one eye. Only the mixture is not so even and stable; it is apt to fall into rival parts. But it can be greatly stabilised by the support of coincident

[1] This is what certain writers mean by "perception." Contrast the meaning in Chap. XX.

contours, as when two postage stamps of similar die but of different colours are used as the right and left halves of a stereoscopic slide. And in various circumstances, e.g. when the contours of a stereoscopic figure, or partially overlapping surfaces, are done in different colours for either eye, we can see two different colours (even complementaries) at the same (binocular) place at once or one colour " through " the other.[1] If the binocular mixture of colours is to be interpreted in the same way as lustre, we should have to infer that the difference between the uniocular and binocular mixture is not nearly so striking and characteristic when only the colours differ as when the brightnesses of the components differ.

The brightness of binocular vision, as we have seen, is the same as that of either eye singly. When one eye is darkened by having a grey glass set before it, the binocular brightness is about the average of the two contributory brightnesses. This mixture of brightnesses therefore behaves like the binocular mixture of neighbouring colours. But when one eye is very much darkened, the combined field seems to lighten up again (Fechner's paradox). This is really an illusory effect ; for it is due to the complete dominance of the lighter field (the limiting case of retinal rivalry) over the darker one in which the contours of objects have been obliterated.[2] This effect holds also between corresponding parts of the two fields of vision.

When complementary colours are mixed binocularly, the result may contain no trace of colour, especially if supporting contours are provided. Here the difference between uniocular and binocular equations is that in the latter far less is needed of the short-waved component for mixture to white. The mixture is not readily attained especially with saturated colours, and some persons seem to find it more difficult than others. Rivalry is apt to supervene. How this mutual annulment of complementaries is to be explained is not at all evident. Possibly the processes of colour vision are binocularly variable in that sometimes the uniocular components come fully to the stage of sensation in independence of one another, while

[1] Cf. Schumann, *Ztsch. f. Psych.*, 1921, **86**, 253 ff.
[2] S. Dawson, op. cit.

under other conditions there is an earlier physiological interference. We do not know. We lack entirely the psychological insight into colour that might lead us to see how complementaries as sensations could (binocularly) annul one another when brought closely enough into contact. A psychological theory of quality of this kind should surely be possible, and here may be the facts leading towards it. But thus far we are unable to pick out the threads of solution. The senses of taste and smell offer traces of similar mixture.

Similar reflexions are prompted by the facts of binocular colour-contrast. When one eye looks at a white patch on a black background through a blue glass, while the other eye observes it through a grey glass, the latter sees the white surface yellow. Edridge-Green's theory of colour-contrast by relative " estimation " of the quantities of the components of light offers an easy, but fallacious, explanation. A grey patch on a red ground, he thinks, looks green because there is so much more green in the light from the grey patch relatively to the red in that light (white daylight being a mixture of all wave-lengths) than there is in the light of the ground which is so loaded with red. " And if an eye is exposed to light while the other is being dark adapted, the latter after three quarters of an hour is only half as sensitive to light as it would have been if both eyes had been dark adapted."[1] The physiological relations connecting the two fields of vision seem both complex and obscure.

In comparison with these vanishing traces of an integration of quality, the integration of the attributes of extent-position is rich and progressive. It is evidently full and systematic, showing no gaps that experimental research may not be expected to fill out satisfactorily. Only on the basis of systemic form is the evolution carried beyond what Table 3 shows. The complication of time stops short at the first stage, not, we may suppose, because time is incapable of further integration, but merely because it is given to us primarily in so limited scope that material is lacking for further advance. We have only one small

[1] C. Behr, *Arch. f. Opthalm,* 1910, **75**, 201 ff, quoted from *Psych. Bull.*, **9**, 101.

(unidimensional) field of time. In fact we may now surmise that the rest of the cognitive mind evolves or builds itself out of and upon the basis given chiefly by the systemic attributes.

Many psychologists have dealt with the mind on the presupposition that the intellect was waiting within it, so to speak, to notice and to elaborate the sensations presented to it. But it is generally unintelligible how any agent such as the intellect or the self could be posted ahead of creation as it were, waiting and watching for the stuff of sensations to appear and able to pack it into parcels and fabricate it into marketable presentations. The principles of science lead us rather to expect that the intellect itself should emerge out of the simpler forms of experience by their complication. It is now often admitted, after the prolonged discussion that has taken place, that some part at least of what the intellect was once thus supposed to do, must be set down to the native processes of sensory complication. The intellect cannot make of three things a star even in art : the three things make the star merely when the intellect gives them a chance. And this chance they get of themselves in the chaos and turmoil of sense without the help of the intellect at all. The world of sense is so constituted that it goes on forming stars all the time. And the stars once formed help to increase the chances of other stars forming, just as we find in the chemical and biological spheres that the more complicated and later units are borne by the earlier and simpler. The active world is slowly brought to birth, but all the reactions its later children exert upon the matrix that bore them should not lead us to suppose that even in mind this natural order is reversed.

CHAPTER XVI

MIND AND ACTION

IN dealing with stereoscopic vision we were forced for the first time to refer frequently to the movements of the sense-organ under the influence of the stimulus. The ear is fixed immovably in the head, and is in so far passively subject to every stimulus that reaches it. But the eye is constantly being drawn from one stimulus to another. Under the guidance of higher processes like attention and interest it even seems in the adult to seek out actively the objects of its own desire. And the two eyes are somehow kept together in the most delicate co-ordination. It therefore behoves us now to consider the relation of mind to bodily action.

But we must first be quite clear and precise about one general principle. We are not going to try to explain the integration of experience by any appeal to external processes, whether they be physiological or psychical. This principle has been firmly established for us by our discussion in the previous chapter. Ensuing movement is doubtless of great importance for physiological integration. One eye sees a bright object, and adjusts itself so that the light from it reaches the fovea. So does the other eye too. In the nervous system these two changes constitute one process, having two points of ingress, two of egress, and one complex of co-ordination between them. The singleness of vision then surely has some relation to this central co-ordination. Undoubtedly! We have that fact already before us in the singleness of our vision. But what we know of the physiological process does not help to explain the singleness of vision. It is our duty to correlate this singleness with the neural integration and to search constantly for new points of parallelism between them. But no explanation accrues therefrom. We should never be so foolish as to suppose that psychical unity would explain or account for a unity on the physical side that we could not fully describe and explain in purely physical terms. That would run counter to the established principles of the physical sciences. In other words, we should be unable to accept any such hypothesis because we should feel it was unsatisfactory, as scientists before us have all felt it to be. Similarly we psychologists must clear our conscience and recognise that any explanation of psychical unity by reference to physiological co-ordination when we cannot properly describe and explain that unity in psychological terms is just as unsatisfactory. Therefore we leave it at that. We recognise psychical unity when it occurs: we recognise its autonomic nature; we describe it as best we can, along with its correlations and dependence on other psychological facts. And we await the light that comes of the progressive classification of these facts. Meanwhile we try to keep in touch with the neighbouring facts of physiological research and classification. But the mind is not therefore, as the philosophy of it has so often suggested, merely a speculative instrument, given to man that he may form for himself a disinterested knowledge of the world, create and enjoy works of art, and plan an elysium of happiness and love. The mind is truly capable of reaching towards these great ideals; but its first purpose is to serve the ends of action.

And the mind is not solely human and adult. There is also undoubtedly mind in the child and the animal. And the adult human mind that we so properly revere surely includes much, if not all, that is typical of the mind of child or animal.

Of course we can only observe our own experiences, never those of any other creature. Our knowledge of the minds of others is based solely upon their actions, whether these be expressions, gestures, movements, words, or any other such bodily events. We are commonly said to infer from these the experiences we attribute to others. And there can be no doubt that this is a correct *logical* description of the process. As such we may let it stand for the present without any enquiry into its validity as a psychological theory.

Physiology has taught that much of our behaviour is purely mechanical. It goes on just as well when we are asleep as when we are awake. Some of it goes on for some time after death (peristalsis, for example). But even when we are awake, doing things of our own accord and freely, much of what we seem to do is really done for us by neural machinery. We go to visit a friend, for example, just to pass the time pleasantly, and we walk some distance to his house. We choose our path carefully, for the road is wet and muddy; and then we see him from afar and greet him with all our attention. What keeps our legs properly in motion when we are so engaged? And while our attention was free, why did we need only to think where to put down our feet in the mud and not how to bring each foot forward to be put down? Machinery, is the answer. We merely helped to modify by sight and judgment a process that was going on by itself and that would plant a foot in the middle of a nasty puddle if we did not judge quick enough.

So mind and mechanism interact, it would seem. In us there is quite a deal of mind; in some animals there is probably none. Wherever there is any mind at all, it doubtless enters into the process of action to the extent of its capacities. How? That is the crucial question. And a very difficult one. No definite answer can be given to it. But we can state the assumptions and hypotheses upon which knowledge seems best to progress.

We have already briefly discussed the idea that the mind responds to certain kinds of neural activity as a whole, in a unique and perfectly inexplicable way that has little or no relation to the nature of the neural activity that prompts it. This theory is neither definite nor useful in the progress of knowledge, and so may be ignored. There are two other hypotheses. Both of them involve the assumption that the mind consists solely of its experiences, and that these experiences are to some extent or other dependent upon "parallel" neural processes. The two hypotheses differ in their idea of the extent or completeness of the parallelism. In the one, psychophysical action is supposed to consist first of an afferent physiological part or series, then of a psychical part set up by

the end of the first series and running on by itself for some time and distance, so to speak, and, lastly, of a final physiological series ending in more or less explicit movements. According to this theory the train of experiences intervenes between two trains of physiological events and connects them. Without it they would not be connected and the final response could not happen. The psychical series is therefore real or independent, at least once it is started, and genuinely active.

Now this theory holds a rather risky and dangerous position. It seems to challenge physiology to produce a continuous series of physiological events leading from stimulus to response, and to imply that it somehow knows physiology cannot do so. This à priori knowledge presumably rests upon our sense of the " reality " of mental activity and effort. If we did not try, things would not happen : therefore the trying is an essential link in the process that can have no physiological parallel. For if it had, we might dispense with trying and the event would still take place.

The physiologist quite properly refuses to accept any such à priori instruction from a discipline external to his own. He will form his own principles on his own data by light of his efforts to bring them into systematic order. And he has now settled down to the assumption that every sort of organic activity, whether it have any psychical counterpart or not, can ideally be displayed as a continuous series of physical events, fully determined according to physical laws. All the extensive and rapid progress of his research supports him in this assumption, which therefore increasingly partakes of the nature of a principle. All the knowledge of experiences that the psychologist can ever produce will never detract one iota from its validity. For being psychological this knowledge has no bearing on it whatever.

But everyone now agrees that experience is dependent upon the stimulation and activity of the nervous system. And it has been shown that injury or defect of the nervous system may supervene at any point in the course of neural activity, and may produce a block or hiatus in any part of the dependent mental processes. We have therefore no other course than to conclude that experience is at every point dependent upon physiological processes.

From these facts many thinkers feel compelled to infer that experiences are not really active processes that cause one another. They are rather merely the shadows that are thrown by the active processes of the brain, an appearance passively attached to these processes, i.e. an epiphenomenon. You look for some time at a blue patch on a grey field, and then look away at another grey field. The blue patch is then replaced by a yellow one, and for some time there is a coming and going of blue, grey, and yellow in that area. But the blue sensation does not cause the yellow one and that the next one. A blue sensation could not cause anything at all as far as we know. Quite true! But the neural processes on whose occurrence the blue sensation probably depends does not by itself alone cause the process that evokes the yellow sensation either. The material basis of it possibly changes under certain influences into the material basis for yellow. Possibly the psychical stuff of blue changes also into that of yellow: we do not know, because we do not yet understand blue and yellow psychologically. That is just the point. Until we do understand our experiences, their inner nature or stuff and its changes, connexions, and complications, we have no right to make assertions about the activity or causal efficacy of experiences, one way or the other. We have certainly no à priori reason to assume that mind is an inert panorama of shadows. Besides, the descriptive aspects of any process, whether it be physical or not, never could cause one another. It is often said that causation in the physical world resolves itself finally into descriptive sequences which reveal to us nothing whatever of any causes or forces that make these sequences what they are. Even quantitative continuity or equivalence would therefore be no sign of a persistent cause. If this is strictly true of physics, we need not despair for psychology. We can expect to discover typical descriptive sequences in experiences too, and to trace out some threads of persistence and equivalence. If epiphenomenalism means that experiences lie inertly and incoherently beside one another while they last, we know from our study of integration and from our common sense that that is false. Our own minds strike us as being full of interconnected parts, to have an inner continuity or sense in them, however ragged and disconnected they may often be, and however little we understand this inner sensibility as yet. Science is said to portray the physical world as a mere mechanism, i.e. devoid of inner sense or coherence. Psychologists do sometimes paint a similar picture of the mind, but at the first glance we see that the thing is a caricature. The conglomerates of sensation that are given out as the analysis of a memory or an idea or a sentiment are no more true than are the familiar futurist pictures of a peasant smoking his pipe or of a country village that looks like a pile of house-breaker's rubbish seen from above. They are impressions, dissections, or syntheses, as you like it; but they are not what they claim to be. You have only to invert the proposition and to ask: is this rigmarole of sensations a memory or an affection? And you see at once that it is not. It is mind with the sense of it destroyed.

We do not therefore need to discuss whether mind creates energy convertible into motion or radiation of any kind. No notion of mental energy or even of mental inertia has yet been established that is of this quantitative nature. And yet we know of no reason why such notions should not be set up for mental processes or for the flow of experiences, or why they should not be set into parallel or equated with the quantitative processes of physics and physiology.

But even if we confine our attention for the present to formulating the probable outlines of psychophysics generally, it is certainly very difficult to see how mind is woven into the mechanism of the nervous system. One of the great difficulties has been created by the results of modern physiological research. This has shown that the neural counterpart of mind, the tracts that run from impression to response through the higher levels of the nervous system serve only to control and regulate or to *condition* far more stable and enduring connexions between impression and response that run through the lower and lowest levels of the nervous system. It therefore appears that these higher tracts (or mind) really of themselves initiate and carry out *nothing*, even though they sometimes seem to do so, as when the automatic underlying reflex actions have been long inhibited or as when they themselves (" we ") release the stimulus that evokes such reflexes.

When food is put into a dog's mouth, the stimulation of skin-senses and of taste excites the flow of saliva in virtue of the inborn reflex connexions that exist between these stimuli and the salivary response. No such inborn connexion attaches to the sense of smell or hearing or sight. But if the dog is fed for some time regularly to the accompaniment of a stimulus on one of these senses, that stimulus acquires (through higher neural tracts) a connexion with the original salivary reflex. Thus afterwards the accompanying stimulus is able alone to evoke a flow of saliva. The dog's mouth waters at the smell or sight of the food, or at the sound thus associated with it. But if this conditioning stimulus is given too often alone, it soon loses its power to excite any flow: the connexion with the primary reflex is lost and dissipated. Therefore the accompanying stimulus is only a modifying condition of a primary mechanism whose presence is an antecedent necessity. And this relation applies to the whole of the higher nervous system, i.e. to the mind in relation to all action of the organism.

It may therefore even seem to be a matter of indifference whether the dog (or man) has any sensations of his food or not. The only requisite is that the conditioning stimulus should strike into the salivary (or other) reflex arc. If afferent nerves at the same time carry excitations to the cortex and evoke sensations there, what difference will they make to his actions? Well, being themselves again accompanying stimuli (or excitations) they will presumably also find their way out into the salivary reflex process, and will therefore be able to modify it. Do we not find that the mere thought of sour things makes the mouth water? All experiences, therefore, in virtue at least of their underlying physiological basis will act as conditions of such actions as the reflex equipment of the body provides and submits to modification by accompanying processes.

In reflecting on this general relation between mind and action we must be careful to maintain the true perspective. We must not exaggerate the functions of reflex processes at the expense of those of mind or conversely. The reflex equipment of the body is not an inert machinery lying ready for any impulses the mind may send it, but otherwise dead-beat. It is full of activity of its own, and if the mind does not give it an opportunity of exercise in due season it will take one itself out of season. Until then it is a power-centre with its own limits of use, fatigue and energy which the mind does well to know familiarly. Within these limits the mind is free to direct its actions.

On the other hand, the mind does direct its actions. If the attention is suddenly arrested, reflex mechanisms like walking are forthwith interrupted. A mind of low grade is not able to put forth more than a fraction of the energy that an intelligent man can exert muscularly, unless it is thoroughly roused by passion or fear. And the neural machinery of mind is itself a part of the whole power installation. The forces which run through it are as really forces as those that work the generator or the dynamo. Every activity of the nervous system is itself autonomous. And conditioning stimuli do make saliva flow when there is no stimulus to the primary reflex. To that extent they really do initiate action and carry it through, i.e. they can do so once they are properly set up, though not absolutely from the beginning. From the genetic point of view it is therefore correct to say that mind initiates nothing, it only allows that to happen at its own time more or less which the body is already prone to. But from the general point of view, for any present moment, the mind, on the contrary, initiates and carries through actions far more truly than does the reflex system. For it does, or allows (according to its relative conditioning force at the moment), whatever suits it and what would not happen then at all but for it. At the same time it has the superior advantage of being able to change its grip upon reflex mechanism—in order the better to regulate its work. It may not lose its hold upon the mechanism or the latter will act blindly and senselessly. But in the affairs of human organisation, which form a cosmos of grades like that of the brain, we always say that work is initiated and carried through by the man who conceives its plan and organises it, although he could do nothing at all without countless workers to achieve it. Of course we are not now making a distinction between the rôle played by different parts of the mind in the initiation of action, e.g. by feeling as against thought.

It should be noticed, however, that this directive force of mind does not primarily imply any sort of teleology, as we find it expressed in the logical formulation of our various actions. There the end of an action is stated abstractly and separately from the means that lead to it and from the motives and forces that prompt it. But there can be no doubt that mental action works just as much from behind under the impulsion of forces as physical action does. Even an end itself, when it is conceived, is a force propelling us in a certain direction, recalling ideas that may serve as means, adhering to one of these more than to another, and so moving or driving forwards to a conclusion or last mental state. Of course the laws by which a mental state drives forward are mental laws, not physical ones. But nevertheless it is true that an idea can no more stand ahead of its own activity or bridge a distance without means of continuity than can any physical power. We can say if we like that all mental action is teleological in so far as there is always some inner sense or coherence binding successive states together, if the action is mental, and not merely physiological with an irregular mental accompaniment. But this must never be interpreted as if the end of the action were there before the beginning or as if coherence somehow worked from the state about to come towards the one that just is. That would be absurd and impossible.

CHAPTER XVII

THE GENERAL SCHEME OF APPETITIVE ACTION

HAVING thus cleared the ground for a study of the mental side of action, we may now consider briefly the typical form of the commonest and most fundamental kind of mental action. This is the work of the appetites. In reflex action the response is elicited within the ordinary range of circumstances whenever the stimulus is applied. There are refractory periods, which are often determined by conditions that proceed from other stimuli: or they may be set by internal stimuli. But in either case these stimuli are limited in range and peculiar to the action in question. They act directly upon the mechanism of the reflex from its original foundation throughout: they do not need to be learnt, and they do not arise subsequently: and if they do so arise as "conditioning stimuli," as in the experiment with the dog, they are not essential to the reflex action.

But there is a large class of actions, to which the co-operation of reflex mechanism is essential, that are periodic and irregular, apparently dependent upon hidden internal circumstances. These are the appetites. An animal will not eat everything put before it at any time, even though the food be palatable. It must have some appetite for the food. The same condition is found in other activities, such as drinking, resting, sleeping, playing, and mating in all its forms and stages. These actions seem to involve the whole organism: they are not wholly preformed, but have largely to be learnt and built up from a simple inborn rudiment: and they seem to involve the mind or experience of the animal. We call them appetites, because the organism seems to seek out what it wants or to be drawn to that object. They are often called instincts: but this term is very vague and has been used so variously and so erroneously that it is better to avoid it. Instinct means "endowed": the animal is fitted out with some mechanism carrying him on in a certain line of action. It is safer to use the word in this sense for the details of the machinery by which the object of the appetite rouses and urges the organism forwards in a certain way. Thus used the term is perhaps a sort of shield for the psychologist's ignorance: the use of the physiologist's term "reflex" would imply that we can specify exactly the reflex process involved at any point—which we are often unable to do. But we must study all forms of actions as far as we yet know them. And instinct will temporarily fill the gap in our knowledge, implying a complex of mechanisms involving stimuli, connexions, and responses upon which appetitive or other types of action are based. So when we say an organism does anything by instinct we shall mean that for the moment it is being carried forwards by some inborn machinery not the result of learning—in a direction not anticipated or foreseen and without any knowledge of the end of its action.

Now it is our concern to study the experiences that accompany or take part in appetitive action. They fall into three parts. First, there are all the sensations that come from the exteroceptive senses: these sensations are dependent upon the external environment of the body in general, and in particular upon the object of the appetite or upon the situation surrounding or preceding the appearance of the object. Then there are the proprioceptive sensations which furnish an awareness of the animal's own limbs and body and their relative postures and movements. Lastly, we have the interoceptive sensations that are dependent upon the inner environment of the body, as it were, and that represent the state of the bodily economy or of the subjective world in its psychically lowest form. They include sensations of hunger, thirst, lust, fatigue, freshness, sleepiness and the like, a group that is not always descriptively distinct from the senses of the other groups. But this tripartite grouping is not supposed to be descriptively exact, but rather functionally important.

The three groups may be briefly described as object, agent, and subject-sensations.

Reflex actions of the simplest kinds probably involve only the action of a single momentary stimulus upon a preformed receptor and its attached transmittor and effector mechanisms. Actions of a more complicated or serial nature, especially during the process of learning or of readjustment, involve stimuli from the agent limbs to regulate their course. Adjuvant and inhibitory forces may accrue from interlocking mechanisms using the same transmittors or effectors, or they may be attached to the reflex mechanisms by associative learning. But the third group of sensations represent a distant and distinct focus of impressions whose stimuli are usually present and continuous in action or absent for much longer periods than those of the other two groups, as hunger, lust, and sleepiness are.

Consequently they partake far more of the nature of aches, urges or stresses than of momentary striking stimuli. They are, of course, all of them physiologically and psychologically positive: they are not negative as their real counterparts—the absence of food or fluid or mate—logically are. They therefore add to the sum of forces coursing through the nervous system and rouse the creature to increased activity along lines indicated by its bodily and neural inheritance. So they make it move about in its environment more actively. But, of course, they do not at all convey to it what the world holds in store that might satisfy its ache. They only increase the animal's chances of meeting with this satisfying thing by making it move more vigorously, and therefore (by chance again) probably farther afield. No creature comes to life with perfectly evenly distributed dispositions to actions. There are always some lines of action ready for use, and likely to be useful in its earliest environment. But the new-born mammal does in general embody a state of greater random activity under first stress of hunger or cold. Nature, however, has taken care that the creature's first environment will provide an almost certain chance of its finding an object that will still these aches: and, if its random efforts mislead it, maternal instinct will move its parent to rescue it from occasional failure. But in the great majority of cases its own efforts will bring it ease.

Upon contact with the right stimulus the reflex endowment of the creature then takes over the action: the sucking process begins with repeated jerking forwards of the head, and, as soon as chance again gives success, the teat is held firmly by the mouth while sucking proceeds; or the offspring, feeling the warm surface of the body, presses forwards underneath so as to attain the greatest area of contact and warmth sensations. These are the circumstances then in which accompanying stimuli acquire connexion with these inborn reflex rudiments of action and so establish themselves as conditioning stimuli. On the recurrence of the ache the reflex mechanism will be the more prone to excitation by its own primary stimulus.

But there is a process of extension of the action on the motor, as well as on the sensory side. This has been clearly displayed by experiments on animal training, in which the work of Thorndike on cats affords a standard pattern. Thorndike enclosed hungry cats in boxes of a special make, which could be opened only by a certain movement or procedure on the part of the enclosed cat. Perhaps a certain bar had to be pressed outwards or a bolt to be depressed or a string to be pulled by a loop: or perhaps the cat had merely to turn and lick its back—it is immaterial which. The cat became very excited upon seeing food outside the cage, rushed towards it, trying to squeeze out between the bars of the cage, jumping up, clawing and scratching. All this represents the heightened activity produced by the inner ache, that is largely of a random character, although in the adult animal there is always plenty of sensible action that has been acquired in its previous experience. Only, in the new environment of the box, that action is almost wholly useless. The animal is then thrown back on chance for its success: and after a variable time, on the average rather long, it does by chance stumble through the action that opens the box. So it reaches the food. On successive trials of this process, the time from the insertion of the cat in the box till the opening of it becomes at first rapidly, and then slowly, shorter on the average. Finally, the cat proceeds calmly and rapidly to open the box without any irrelevant action at all.

The progress of learning in animals has been very frequently studied with the help of mazes, of which the Hampton Court maze is a familiar type. Minute observation is kept on the behaviour of the animal from its first entry into the maze till it is able to run through it without error. When the animal enters a blind alley it may run to the end of it or only a little way along it ; and on returning from it, it may retrace the maze to some extent or continue by the correct route. Peterson [1] found that the progress of learning brings a rapid decrease in the proportion of retracing movements and the exploration of a blind alley is progressively reduced till it is eliminated. Accordingly when a blind alley is shortened, it is eliminated more quickly. And De Camp [2] has shown that rats learn readily to choose the shorter of two (separate) paths to food with a threshold difference of one in ten. This suggests that learning takes place simultaneously throughout the course that has to be learnt.

In learning to get out of one of Thorndike's boxes, an animal obviously does not learn by repeating a single series of movements, as we learn the alphabet, from beginning to end. For in the end all the random scrambling and turning is eliminated. And only one action is common to every chance success, namely, that which actually opens the box or makes the experimenter open it. This suggests to us that the progress of learning may here be by retroactive, rather than by successive, associations. And Vincent [3] found in maze experiments that the blind alleys in the second half of the maze tend to be eliminated before those in the first half. But other experimenters have not been able to agree with these conclusions. The process of learning in these mazes is far more complicated than would seem at first glance. And perfect backward elimination would probably only take place if the final satisfaction were the sole agency in favouring and fixing associations. The tendency to retrace the maze for some

[1] *Behav. Monog.*, 1917, **3**, No. 15.

[2] *Psychobiol.*, 1920, **2**, 245 ff.

[3] *J. An. Behav.*, 1915, **5**, 367 ff.

distance would unduly increase the work with the earlier blind paths. Besides this factor of frequency there is also the vividness of impression that may ensue from all sorts of accidental and inherent circumstances of action, the special details peculiar to parts of the journey and the differences between long unimpeded runs and those that are soon checked by alleys, etc.

And animal learning involves not only the learning of what is learnt, but the inhibition of what is not adopted. It can be induced not only by results that appeal to appetites, but also by effects that might arouse repellent emotion (pain or punishment of some kind or other). Such inhibition appeared in Thorndike's experiments when animals that had been taught to take a roundabout way to freedom, did so even when the obstructing wire was removed. And it has been re-discovered in Köhler's experiments on responses learnt to the brighter of two simultaneous signs : even when the weaker was replaced by one still stronger than the other, the response was to this strongest one. The part played by such inhibition must help to create a unitary whole in any complex action : but it is very difficult, of course, to prove the presence of such wholes experimentally, except by this kind of inference and by the fact that the animal improves its action on the whole from one trial to the next, progressing in learning and inhibition simultaneously. But the presence of wholes becomes more evident with increasing intelligence of the learner. It is particularly evident as soon as there is any sign of constructive ability, creating means of reaching distant positions by devices that have not hitherto been employed. The chimpanzee [1] and the human infant at an early stage display this kind of understanding clearly.

Thus we see how action extends under the stress of an inner urge, partly by extension of the receptive basis of the action into conditioning stimuli and partly by extension of the effector side of the action into conditioning movements. In adult life action may thus become so complex that we can hardly believe it ultimately rests upon such a limited and primitive rudiment as can exist

[1] W. Köhler, *Abh. Preuss. Akad.*, 1918, Ph. M. Klasse. No. 2. *Psych. Forsch.*, 1922, 1 ff., *The Mentality of Apes*, 1925.

in the new-born. The extension of the receptive process amplifies and elaborates the object of the action: the motor extension increases the part played by the agent in the process. At every moment the animal must be held to its work by the inner stress: it must be held to the object by external sensory stimuli: and it must be able to regulate its movements to the action of the latter by data that represent the position of its limbs at any moment. Of course these last do not need to become conscious at every moment, any more than they do in our experience of walking. But they must be capable of becoming conscious in so far as the creature is to modify them ("control" them) in accordance with its sensory experiences: i.e. in so far as they are correlated with changes of conscious experience.

Of course it is impossible to rationalise the entry of mind into action: for we can always in principle rationalise the action of an organism in the quantitative terms of energetics, at least with approximate completeness. The lower forms of action are undoubtedly completely mechanical. But as conditioning processes increase, we come nearer and nearer to action that involves experience. Any experience seems generally to be bound up with action as a complex condition of it: not merely as a trivial accessory condition, modifying it slightly when it is otherwise elicited; but as a condition that even in the simpler forms of action is capable of acting for a short time at least as a complete condition, like the accompanying stimulus that is able alone to excite some flow of saliva. And this power no doubt grows greater and greater until it will work over long periods and with great force.

Purely reflex action does not seem to involve any factor of the cumulating, stressing, nature of the urges or appetites. So we might venture to look upon appetitive action as the lowest form of action that involves experience. Possibly this tripartition is characteristic of all mind-controlled action. The higher forms of such action seem to differ, not in introducing new groups of factors, but in the degree of complication and integration of the experiences within each group. In appetitive action the urge is a mere sensation: in the action of an intelligent mammal it may be introduced by a series of preceding conditions that tend to obviate its cruder stresses and to prepare for its appearance: or in man it may grow into a sense of duty towards the needs of others. The growth of the object is familiar in the study of cognition: to a pig it is the root he encounters in digging; to a man it is the seed that will one day grow into a tree bearing fruit. The increase of our hold on movement is also familiar. The child learns golf by trial and practice, but the studious adult learns to analyse the movements of the game into many special parts, to any of which a slight change may be consciously imparted for some special purpose. This analytic, conceptual control of movement is possibly harder to attain than is the complication of the other two factors.

Our study of action shows us finally how little of our action is preformed. We are prepared to respond to certain simple stimuli in certain simple ways, but we have no foreknowledge, as it were, of the objects of our environment and of how to act towards them. We have to form in our impressions or in our minds by the force of associative stimulation (and the ensuing integration of experience) the objects of our world, and we have to mould our action to their nature. So we are prepared to meet almost any environment that comes within the scope of our generalised rudiments of inborn action.

The kitten, for example, is not born with a foreknowledge of mice and their ways and shapes. But it is endowed with nervous organisation that compels it to run after moving things, even dancing shadows and sunbeams. If now, on grabbing at the moving "thing" with claws and teeth, this behaves as a mouse does, has to be held firmly, escapes, runs, has to be held firmly again, and when bitten tastes pleasant, then the kitten will eat it. So an association of some strength is formed. When repetition has made this strong enough, the kitten will not merely run after a mouse, but will run towards the smell or sound or sight of one. But a kitten that has had no experience of mice will respond to none of these impressions. In the course of time the kitten not only responds to impressions remotely connected with mice, but it also acquires modes of action suitable for each stage of approach towards the actual mouse, e.g. search (random at first, then by association growing "clever"), patient waiting, postures for springing, teasing play, carrying the mouse to its young, etc. Kittens thus fed by the parent learn early to associate the smell and sound and form of mice with one another and so become mousers.

Nevertheless, at a certain stage of life, usually about the second month, the kitten is more responsive to its first experience of a mouse than at any earlier or later time. It bristles up its hair; it switches its tail; it may hiss, spit, or growl; it catches the mouse by the back of its neck. Whether these mechanisms are emotional in origin, like our goose-flesh, trembling, cries and the many unapparent changes in states of fear and rage, we do not know. But they are doubtless likewise the effect of some such simple cause upon a series of inherited response-mechanisms. They do not in any sense imply that the kitten has any sort of psychical predisposition for mice. It still has to fit its experience on to the mechanisms it inherits in more or less detail and to adjust the latter to the needs of the former.

Neither cat nor dog are born hereditary enemies prepared with a malicious forehatred of one another. They are always enemies by discovery of each other's ways, whereby they also discover themselves. They are so differently constituted that, if they once meet by accident they will inevitably annoy one another, just as oil and water by nature fail to mix. There is little harm, of course, in speaking of foreknowledge and such things in a general practical way, but any such carelessness of expression may be very misleading psychologically, admitting to our science the most fantastic hypotheses. It is for this reason that we must distinguish so carefully between mechanisms ready to be excited in a simple summary way and the ensuing adaptations between associated stimuli and modifications of mechanical response.

Thus the senses at birth are quite unconnected fields. This must not, however, tempt us to suppose that the field of any one sense is then still undifferentiated, as many have supposed, or is all in confusion. Music that passes unheeded is just as orderly and coherent as any that is eagerly heard. The sunset is all there for the puppy, just as much as it would be for a man whose colour vision was of the same scope as the puppy's, whatever that may be. The difference lies not in the sense itself, but in the way the other mental activities of the listener are interlinked in an orderly manner with the sensations that form the elements of the music or of the sunset. We have to learn to find our way about in the sounds we hear; but they already contain all the differences and relations that we can ever learn to detect and to follow in them. The sunset does not appeal to the puppy because it does not enter into alliance with any urge or need of his. It becomes the basis of no current of activity.

CHAPTER XVIII

SENSORY SPACE IN GENERAL

WE are now free to follow out the further course of the integration of experience. We have considered how mind is related to action, and we have recognised clearly that this relation does not explain the integration of mind at all. We must study that integration descriptively and positivistically, not looking for any explanation of it from without its own range. So our next task is to look for and study the complication of sense that comes after the third dimension of forms, realised for us in stereoscopy. This complication will be more inclusive than that elaboration of a single sense: but, as no single sense shows any greater elaboration than stereoscopy, we may expect to find that different senses are involved in the next stage of elaboration. That seems the step required to continue the series: particle of sensation, aggregation of these particles in a single field, two fields of the same sense. From our previous analysis we should further expect to find that the forms of different senses should combine to constitute a more inclusive unifying form, which the contributory forms help to produce and sustain without thereby losing their own identity.

It has often been held, and is commonly held still, that all the senses are spatial from the first. That is implied in the recognition of an attribute of localisation. It is also the criticism that has usually been urged against Kant, who propounded the theory that space is a "form" supplied by the mind and applied by it to the data of sense—the elements of sensation. For, he argued, the (logical) mind cannot make space out of the non-spatial aspects of sensation by some subtle chemistry of its own; and if you say one sensation is already beside another, you have therewith presupposed this spatiality. Therefore space is something more than is the datum of sense ; and as it is not so much a datum of any sensation as a unitary whole that includes and contains all sensations, it must have come from some other source than sensation, i.e. presumably from the mind itself.

And we have from the outset recognised that localisation cannot be an attribute of any single particle of sensation. For it involves a reference from one sensation to other experiences concerned with the same point of space. Localisation just means this reference to experiences that share this location : and each one is localised by indication of the others thus correlated with it. The elementary particle of sensation, or the aggregates of them that we find in the field of any one sense, possess only the attributes of position and extent. Whatever variations of these they include, constitute, at the most, extents, distances, forms, motions, and the like, but never spatial structures of any kind.

We have also rejected the idea that localisation could be founded solely upon differences in the quality and intensity of sensations, as has frequently been maintained. Not only are the variations of these attributes that occur too limited to account for the great range of localisation, but we can see no affinity between the essence of localisation and these qualitative attributes. Besides, if an "attribute" of localisation did appear along with these bundles of qualitative and intensive differences, it would have to be something over and above them : and, therefore, we should be unable to escape the more economical inference that it merely occurred along with them and was not produced by them in any way. Then we should be back again at our nativistic position. And as we do not actually find bundles of qualitative and intensive differences bereft of all attributive position, even under special experimental conditions, we have no reason at all to suppose that these differences produce the positional attribute. Kant's opposition to this genetic line of argument was concerned with the conceptual manipulation of data that had no spatial features. We could not, he held, by conceptual thought extract any notion of space from sensory data that were utterly unspatial: therefore space must be primarily a property of sense. His next step was to show that it could not be property of the crude stuff of sensation —its elements, as we should say.

We do not follow him in denying position to the elements of sensation: these have an attribute in virtue of which one is beside a second and not beside a third: or in virtue of which they constitute extents at one region of a sensory field and not at another. But we agree with him as soon as "neighbourhood" refers to the elements of different senses. As soon as you say a touch is at or near a place that you see, you are postulating a medium in which they both stand, and which is neither the surrounding field of touch nor that of vision. And as this new medium is itself a continuous and therefore single "whole," it must be something over and above the raw stuff of sensation. To call it a "whole" does not, of course, imply that it is always present as a whole.

It did not occur to Kant to suggest that this new medium was the self-synthesis of the raw material of sense it seems to be applied to and to envelop. The new medium was a form of "intuition" (sensory experience, as we should say) supplied by the mind, lying implicitly ready in wait in the mind. It thus becomes difficult to see why it should take upon itself to envelop the raw stuff of sensation. Is it not more reasonable to look upon the new aspect as an integrate emerging out of the data it synthesises and upon whose differences it rests?

We must, therefore, look upon the different senses as in the beginning non-connected fields. This is certainly most probable for the senses other than those of the skin. It alters nothing in our view, of course, that any sense may be reflexly bound up with movement and thereby with the articular sense. For as we have seen, such reflex attachments do not imply the occurrence of accompanying experiences. And even when the experiences supervene as accompanying conditions, each will primarily act as a condition by itself. Being conditions of the same reflex does not imply any special kind of synthesis between them as sensations. That synthesis will itself have to appear, and may thereupon act in turn as a new condition. Why it appears is for the sciences of psychophysics to say, each dealing with its own side of the process and then aligning their results.

The means of correlation of sensory fields is suggested by the parallel problem in stereoscopic vision. Similar changes of position and extent as well as of their integrative complexes constantly occur in a number of sensory fields. A child moves its rattle about in its hand and at the same time sees it move through similarly varying distances, at similarly varying speeds, etc. Not that an articular distance is equal to some visual one: that seems beyond our power of observation to assert until we have established equality by the ensuing correlation. But articular magnitudes vary in size by just noticeable or equal or irregular steps of certain grades while visual magnitudes vary similarly in relation to one another. These parallel changes surely provide a basis for correlation of the two senses.

When the fields of various senses have been correlated in this way, any distance in one comes to be the equivalent of a distance in any other. Or rather, it takes on a new character; from having been a mere distance in its own sense, it becomes a distance-space or simply a space. To put it tersely, mere form becomes space. The tri-dimensional forms of stereoscopic vision become spatial volumes or solids. Binaural positions become the localisation of sounds. A tactual position becomes a tactual localisation—a touch at a spot that the eye can see and the finger reach. All the fields of the senses thus become parts of an inclusive field—sensory space—which has been built up out of the several sensory fields in so far as they present positions, distances, and forms that are similar and vary together. Space is the product of their integration; it is at once their bond and their container, adding to them so as to knit them all together and yet leaving each one unimpaired.

Let us look back and compare for a moment this state of integration with the one from which it presumably arises. Stimulation of the skin yields a field of touch, a field of warmth, a field of cold, and a field of pain. Each sensation in any one field differs in position from any other sensation in that field, but in the beginning it probably bears no definite relation to the positions that attach to the sensations of other senses.[1] In the end the four fields are coincident for sensation, as it were overlapping or interpenetrating each other completely.

We may recall at this point the discussion of lustre and other qualitative fusions, which seem to imply the occurrence of two or more different qualities of sensation *either* in homogeneous intermixture in a single sensory field (that field consisting probably of a mottled array of qualitatively different particles as in the case of grey) *or* as patches in different fields that have been integratively identified, as in the case of binocular lustre and perhaps in that of heat. The co-ordination of the four skin senses might be brought under either head.

We have seen how important the sense of pressure is in its two " kinds "—passive and active. Skin sense is *par excellence* the field of touch, whose areas are for the most part physically fixed except where they may be relatively displaced at the joints. And there, on opposite aspects of the motion taking place, differences of pressure-tension occur that we learn to correlate with changes of form in vision, with changes of passive-pressure in touch, and so on. And muscular sensations will readily be correlated with active-touches in so far as muscular impulses evoke both of them at once. The eye is in actual measurement a tiny field of stimulation, but its cerebral projection is vast; in the end it is the most inclusive field of all, giving the whole body a position as a mere fragment of its own contents. Similarly, the ear gives the merest fragment of (transverse) extensions for spatial purposes; but its localisations finally refer, though imperfectly, to the whole sphere about the head. Taste and smell are stowed away by their correlation into small surfaces in the space of sense—about the tongue and the nostrils.

[1] It does not seem to be clear whether the cerebral areas for the lower senses are so distinct from one another as they are from those of vision, hearing, taste and smell. But it is known that they are conducted through the spinal cord by different routes. No doubt the cerebral co-ordination of these lower senses with one another and with movement is very favourably prepared in the prenatal brain plan.

All this has often been described by saying that our sensations of sight and sound are projected outwards from the body upon or towards the things they come from, while our skin sensations are only projected as far as the skin. On this hypothesis localisation is supposed to start where the neural process subserving sensation ends—at the cerebral cortex. A theory of this kind seems to imply that we can somehow get out of our minds to the real material things around us (or even to our own brain in the first instance) and so localise our sensations at them. That is plainly a begging of the question, explaining localisation by assuming it as already possible or accomplished (viz. in or upon the brain). Our several senses, on the contrary, remain for ever as they began—orderly fields. Localisation is their correlation. Our touch sensations by themselves are never "at the skin," either primarily or finally; to begin with they merely have a positional attribute in virtue of which they stand at certain distances from other discrete touches occurring at the same moment. When one of these touches becomes correlated with a visual sensation of the finger-tip, which stands in a certain position in the visual field and at certain distances from other visual sensations, the touch-sensation does not suffer any alteration or displacement at all; it is essentially unalterable, just like a chemical element in compounds. But it is correlated in the spatial integration with this finger-sight; these two then refer to one another and together form a point of a new all-inclusive system—space. Then the touch sensation "means" or is this spatial point which the finger-sight and the finger's articular position also "mean." And so the touch is now "in the finger." If this process be called projection, well and good. But one must note carefully that no sensation ever had in itself any other position in the beginning than it now has; only its correlations with other sensations can be altered.

Examples of these alterations are occasionally displayed. The most striking is Stratton's experiment[1] with glasses worn in front of his eyes that inverted the whole system of visual presentations, making really high placed objects

[1] *B. Rev.*, 1897, **4**, 341 ff. 463 ff.

appear in the lower part of the visual field and low placed objects in the high part. The natural inclination that ordinary space habits explain, was to reach the hand up for the objects that seemed to lie high, when, of course, the hand would be seen to be moving in the wrong direction, away from the object intended. But in course of time a new adjustment was acquired, whereby Stratton was prompted to move the hand downwards for a high lying visual object. The learning of "mirror-drawing" provides another instance of this alteration of correlations. We have all thoroughly learnt some of these alterations already: it is, for example, perfectly easy to trace out a star-figure in mirror vision when the figure is laid on the top of one's head! That particular adjustment we have all already learnt in combing our hair before the mirror. Obviously, therefore, intersensual correlations are always very particular adaptations.

This may be seen very clearly by writing a word with one's finger on different parts of one's skin: the written touches will seem to be very variously related to vision, sometimes giving a feeling of being written as seen, at other places of being written reversed or upside down according to the ideal point of visual view that seems to be involved.

By the exception the rule is proved. And we are fortunate in having a very notable exception to the rule just stated.

We have seen how peculiar the sensory field of sound is: enormously long (relatively) in one (longitudinal or musical) dimension, and very short in its other (transverse) dimension that gives a basis for the spatial localisation of the different sounds established in the longitudinal aspect.

Now this longitudinal aspect of the auditory field is never brought into connexion with the tri-dimensional space that results from the integrative correlation of the various senses. Not that there is any lack of variation in it; we have seen how finely differentiated pitch-positions are and how evenly graded are their tonal volume. The physical theory of sound teaches us to connect differences of pitch with the wave-lengths of aerial vibration; but the sense of hearing knows nothing of this. Nor is it the case that the sensory basis of music is wanting in ordinal or positional differentiation or is devoid of mass, volume, proportion and motion. Music is full of these, but they never become spatial motion or volume, etc.; for the clear reason that the (real or physical) spatial values and changes of the sounding body do not produce similar positional or volumic values and changes in the different senses, including the longitudinal aspect of the auditory field. They do so only to the approximate exclusion of the latter. And a body may remain spatially unaltered to the skin, the hand, and the eye, and yet change for this aspect of hearing, namely, when it plays a tune, etc. But when the playing body moves in space, it thereby in many cases alters the values of the (transverse) binaural position-series and this series does become a spatial one.

This reference to the spatial values and changes of the sounding body does not imply an appeal to something outside the mind, something physical, as if that could be a standard and regulator for the activities of mental processes. We must remember that the lowly mind that is still confined within these reaches of sensory integration, has no knowledge at all, and so cannot "have" a physical object before its mind. But, of course, if we accept the results of common knowledge and of science as true, there really is a physical object there acting through the sense organs upon the sensations and making them change with its own changes as far as the functions of the organ allow. These changes in sensation then integrate in any way they can, leading in course of time to that level of mind that can know about the physical world that plays upon the organs of sense. It is difficult for us in thinking about the mind to adopt this objective attitude towards it, because we men actually do know much about the things around us. But it is really as absurd to beg the question continually in this way by implying that we connect sensations together because they are ultimately caused by the same physical object, as it would be to imagine (inversely) that the chemicals in a test-tube react in their ways because they are objects of interest at the same moment to the chemist who holds the tube. We all suppose they react with one another because it is in their nature to do so. Thus, although the physical object (like the chemist) is responsible for the reacting things (sensations) being there at all at that moment, the reactions that ensue amongst them are due entirely to the inherent nature of these sensations themselves (including the variations impressed upon them by their physical causes through psychophysical parallelism).

Nevertheless, as we have seen, the positional basis of the longitudinal (musical) aspect of hearing is fundamentally the same as that of the transverse (localisational) aspect, and as that of the localisational values of the other senses. The basis in each case is variation in the systemic attribute of position. It is for this reason that music, though its component tones do not occupy different points of space, has a *quasi* spatial character, as has often been said. It reveals magnitudes, forms, and movements in a realm (a "space") of its own, a realm that is nowhere, as far as our common space of experience is concerned; or rather it has a "where" all to itself; it borders on our space, we might say, and yet stands in no discoverable orientation to it. Music in a very real sense is the mysterious land of the fourth dimension. And when music floats through the air on the wings of time, it actually revels in the luxury of five (psychical) dimensions.

This peculiar mystery of music—for it has long been felt to be its special character—has earned for the art the claim to be the highest purest art, nearest to the divine. But the musical dimension of positions and volumes, from the psychological point of view, is obviously not any more divine than are the three dimensions we call spatial. It is, indeed, non-material, intangible, invisible. But these spatial dimensions are essentially capable of as much divinity as is the non-spatial realm of music.

After all is said and explained, this apartness of music is a most fascinating and curious feature of our mental constitution that has given hearing amongst the senses quite a peculiar individuality and charm.

CHAPTER XIX

APPARENT SIZE

HAVING thus surveyed the problem of the formation of sensory space in a general way, we may now study it in a special form. One of the most important problems of space is the study of apparent size. This problem is most patent in the sense of vision. Everyone knows that from the top of a very high tower buildings look like dolls' houses and men like creeping insects. But houses in a street or round a square all look their proper size, even when we are not at the same distance from them all. We can easily distinguish roughly between the visual extents of the surfaces we see. And by simply holding up a standard line between the eye and any object we can easily find out exactly how broad the surface is to the eye alone. In doing this we cut the primitive field of vision out of its usual setting in sensory experience, showing up what it gives and preventing its data from getting their usual integrative "meanings." Thus we see that the problem of apparent size is likely to be a part of the problem of space. Other senses show differences of apparent size, but not with anything like the range and patency of vision.

As already indicated the apparent size of a visual object is primarily dependent upon the size of the retinal image of the object. This in turn varies in either dimension inversely with the distance of the thing from the eye. The rules of mathematical perspective are based upon this inverse relation. When we see all the lamp-posts in a long street almost in line with one another, we see how they decrease in apparent size regularly as the distance increases.

But if we look round in turn at each of the lamp-posts within a stone's throw of us, we shall not ordinarily without special effort detect this difference. Under ordinary circumstances we see them all of the same size, whether they are farther or nearer. We could tell at once whether the one fifty yards to the left were shorter or taller by even a small amount than the one that lies twenty yards to the right. So there must be another determinant of apparent size than the retinal image. And it is one that is much less familiar. Although we can all judge equality of size within a certain range of distance in spite of difference of distance, many persons, even artists, are so familiar with the projective measure of size that they refuse to acknowledge this constancy-in-spite-of-distance.

The second factor is the degree of convergence of the two eyes. When the eyes are strongly converged, as when they look at a point near the nose, the object looks proportionately small; when they are weakly converged or when their lines of regard are parallel, as when they look at a far object, the object looks proportionately large; and, for intermediate degrees of convergence the relations are proportionate.

The influence of convergence can readily be demonstrated. In exact experiments the retinal impressions of an object can be kept constant by placing it in the form of a figure drawn on a card upon the circumference of circles concentric with either eye. Thus all degrees of convergence —from the greatest possible (as if the object were almost in front of the nose) to parallel line of regard—can be obtained. A much simpler and quite convincing test can be made by placing two fresh coins of the same die two or three inches apart on an unvariegated background in parallel orientation to one another. A pencil point is held above and between them, and is drawn slowly towards the face until the central two of the four coin images that appear, fuse exactly to one. This one will appear to be the nearer and the smaller the farther apart the coins are for any given distance of the head from the surface they lie on. A penny can thus be made to appear smaller than a farthing. Obviously the distances from either eye to both coins are only slightly different, not nearly so different as they would have to be to explain the change of apparent size by reference to the size of the retinal images. For the fixation p of Fig. 19 they are practically equal to those for a point midway between the two coins, where a single coin looks much larger, namely, the size of a penny.

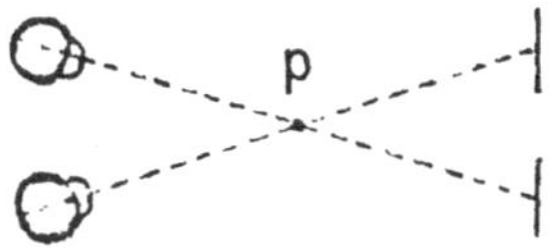

Fig. 19.

These two chief factors determining apparent size thus work against one another. When a thing is near the eye, it makes a large retinal image, and so tends to appear proportionately large, but it requires a strong convergence and so tends to appear proportionately small. Thus over the range of distances that require a distinguishable difference of convergence, things will tend to appear to be of a constant size. Common observation tells us that a person does not appear to swell and shrink in size as we see him walking about in a large room. The plates round a table can all be seen to be equal; and if by some miracle they were all made to suit exactly the sizes of the retinal images they evoked in a spectator, he would see them all just in these different sizes as he looked round the table. They would certainly not look equal to him.

But when the influence of convergence is nil, as when things are very far off or when you look down from a high tower upon a busy street, the moving people seem like specks, strangely unlike any human appearance. Or if you set a number of equally tall people in a row against your eye, you will see them as the photographic camera or the retina does, small in proportion to their distance. Therefore, the photographer must be careful to make his figures and groups stand all in one plane or nearly so. A motor-car shown by the cinema rushing towards you appears to swell interminably, because while the screen-size (like the retinal image) is always properly increasing, your eye does not change its convergence at all, as it would were you actually looking at an approaching car. On the other hand, when you look at your hand with one eye shut, it keeps its size at varying distances, because by fixating it, you make the closed eye take up the proper postures for convergence that would accompany fixation with both eyes. So the constancy of size is not due to the second eye seeing but to the process of converging. But when the one eye keeps a constant posture of fixation, the moving hand seems to swell and shrink in size.

When an after-image is " projected " upon surfaces at different distances from the eye, it appears to have the size that in each case would be proportional to the distance. The primary surface filled a certain angle for each eye and the after-image continues to fill that angle. Its apparent distance depends upon that of the surface it is projected upon and upon the angle of convergence of the eyes. The former gives the relative distances from one another of the things seen, the latter gives the absolute distance of the object fixated, and so sets the scale of proportions for the whole field for that fixation.

Interesting studies of the relation between apparent size and position in the visual third dimension have been carried out in experiments in which two rows of objects running away from the observer had to be set so as to make an apparent *allée*, i.e. so that each object should appear to lie at the same distance from its fellow in the other row. The clearer the depth is shown, the more nearly does the apparent parallel reach the real one. In these parallels the subject attends most to the direction of the lines of depth given by the objects and not to the breadth of the *allée*. Where conditions are so arranged that the apparent *allée* is determined by comparison of the breadth between a pair of objects at varying distances, compared and made equal in each case to a standard distance, the work of attention is quite different. The single objects are sharply fixated and the direction is neglected. The concern of the observer is to see the depth position of the object clearly. Here again the best results approximate to the objective parallel and require great practice as well as the presence of effective criteria for the apprehension of depth positions. The worst results approximate the relations found for the after-image.

Two questions inevitably arise out of these observations : (1) Which is the primary feature—depth-distance or apparent size ? (2) How does convergence bring its influence to bear upon visual forms so as to alter their magnitudes ? In spite of all enlightenment about projective sizes, it remains very difficult to give even an approximately true account of the latter in many cases. Try for instance to draw on paper the perspectival size of the sun or moon. You will draw it far too big. The same difficulty will show itself for any object in the room that is not up against another in your eye. There is surely a "native" element in size that must ultimately rest upon the extents of the retinal image. And by suitable projection upon the retina it is easy to recapture the relations of these sizes. Our study of illusions showed us that magnitudes could be altered by circumstances. The difficulty in vision is the relatively enormous alterations we find that seem to swamp the native magnitudes beyond recognition.

The influence of convergence can probably operate only through the integration of space, otherwise presented or recalled and intended. For vision and optical muscle strain are so entirely different qualities that we can hardly suppose they fuse so closely that we cannot see their togetherness, especially as such close fusion occurs in no other region of sense. And in so far as the influence of convergence upon absolute binocular localisation, e.g. of a single point of light in the darkness, can be isolated, it appears that we are affected by it very little, if at all, in our judgments. Retinal disparity can, of course, be set up between successive impressions, and the least suggestion of it suffices, it would seem. Any traces of difference of brightness are also readily seized for use in estimating distance. We therefore hardly need seriously contemplate any integrational fusion of visual and muscular sensations in this connexion. So we are thrown back upon a purely visual basis. Just as in the change of fixation to right or left, up or down, the amount of the angular change is fixed by the distance we see and attend to, before moving, between the first point of fixation and the second, so in the change of fixation from near to far the distance between these points is either actually present stereoscopically before the change, and is necessarily attended to in order that the change may take place, or it is functionally present in the double images which become the object of attention. An absolute element must, of course, be involved in our awareness of the first point of fixation from which we set out. But a strong basis of absoluteness is always present in the familiarity of the perceptions we usually have and in our collected information about them. When that is absent, as when a wall of fog or a gap in the middle ground or a difference of atmosphere occurs, then our judgment of distance apart from retinal disparity becomes very liable to error.

The question of primacy brings us quickly before the problem of defining the term " absolute " in reference to the positions and magnitudes of sensations. The common-sense view of to-day is coloured chiefly by the simpler physical notions of the immediate past. The positions and magnitudes of sensations would then correspond to the spatial distribution of cerebral excitations and would thereby be rigidly fixed. We do not need to enter into a discussion of the latest problems of relativity in physics in order to see that we can no longer posit any such absolute basis. But relative parallelism may reasonably be admitted. The view that the progress of sensory integration suggests, is that absoluteness is approached by the widening scope of integrative reference. And, in fact, it is itself a product of integration. For, if we had only a single sense, or if a sense remained completely isolated from other senses, as the musical aspects of hearing virtually do, the question of absoluteness of position and magnitude would never arise at all. How could anyone suggest that the pitch of a tone or the magnitude of its volume is a rigidly fixed thing ? This aspect of them has never emerged, we might rather say. All the functions of tones that are given in observable aspects of sensation or in notable products of integration, are entirely independent of any absoluteness of theirs. They set forth only relative position—up, down, between in pitch ; relative magnitude—greater, lesser, equal volumes ; relative proportion—interval of octave, fifth, second ; relative motion—faster, slower, dead melodic passage, etc. For all we know, these values might fluctuate irregularly. But they could not do so singly or in smaller groups without detection.[1] Thus a pitch could not at one

[1] Recent data regarding the functions of the volume of tones, however, do suggest that the volume at any given pitch may be an " absolute " magnitude whose relative fluctuations are " detected " as functions of binaural position. Cf. above, p. 125 note.

moment be raised, so as to make a larger interval with a given tone than at another, without possible detection. And these musical data never come into such integrative correlation with irregularly varying data of other senses as would produce a sense of fluctuating values.

Thus we are justified in speaking of the " real " size of the things we see. A seen thing appears to have a fixed size within a large range of eye movements. This does not mean, of course, that the object is felt to be so many inches broad or high, but merely that it seems sensorially to be of a certain magnitude. A man ten yards off looks his height, as he also does at two or five yards. And for this reason when he is five hundred yards off he appears to be no bigger than your finger perhaps.

So an artist who does not wish to draw like the camera, but desires to give the spectator of his picture the same kind of impression of an interior (i.e. a scene into the ordinary apprehension of which the factor of convergence distinctly enters) must keep real unit sizes nearly the same apparent sizes in his picture. One rule of thumb for interiors says: think all the objects in the room far away from the eye and then enlarge them all proportionately; i.e. if they were fifty yards away they would be relatively so nearly equally distant that unit real size and apparent size would be nearly the same throughout the group; but they would all be too small, hence they have to be enlarged proportionately.

Besides real size, we see real form. The plates lying round a table all look circular, although we see perhaps only the one before us in full face. This has often been discussed, as if the plate never really looked circular except when it was held so that it cast a circular image on the retina. But that statement ignores altogether the third dimension of vision. If a plate is held up before the face and turned on an axis vertical to the line of sight, we keep on seeing its circularity until the line of sight nearly coincides with a diameter of the plate and then again till it has turned through 180° more. If it is turned on a horizontal axis in the frontal plane, we see its circularity only when the plate is vertical, as there is no vertical disparity of retinal images. But we all recognise this lapse of stereoscopy as exceptional and disturbing, when we ever notice it. This we seldom do, because the indications of perspective very often restore the appearance of circularity, as, e.g. with the plates round a table. And eye-movements with their varying accommodation would make up for the lapsed data of vision. The careful tests described above show that perspective yields only apparent solidity (or circularity), not the real thing. Generally a plate looks what it "really" is, circular, not elliptical as the retinal image of it usually is. Its "real" shape, i.e. the shape we commonly see in it, is circular.

There is some evidence that we also see the "real" colours of things. Every artist knows how difficult it is to make the practically minded person see what the artist thinks are the true colours of things, and the latter retorts in his kindlier moods by taking the artist's transcriptions as imaginative idealisations or "interpretations" of nature. But the truth seems wide enough to include both. Each man sees truly. The artist sees perhaps nearer to the retinal colours of the impression ; the practical man sees what the artist in his off-time would probably also call the real colours of the thing, a colour abstraction in which allowance seems to have been made for any unusual illumination, either unusually bright or dull or coloured, etc. It is by this abstraction that we can at once tell whether a thing has changed its colour for some other reason than illumination. But neither the actual process of vision nor the explanation seems yet very clear.

These matters show how very complex vision is and how far we still are from a full knowledge and comprehension of it. The old theory was very simple : "experience" yielded us a knowledge of what was real and what not ; how a man should ever get outside his own mind to gather a knowledge of the real properties of reality was not explained, not lucidly as least. Perhaps the idea was, as has recently been definitely suggested, that when a thing came flat up against the skin, it would impress its real size and form upon the sense of touch. But in touch also we find varying impressions of size from different areas for the same stimulus. Whatever part experience may play in these processes, we can definitely say that any simple interpretation of "experience" is quite inadequate to explain them.

CHAPTER XX

PERCEPTION A SPATIAL FRAGMENT

HAVING traced the progress of integration from the single sensory field through the combined (visual) fields of stereoscopy to the field of space, to which all the senses contribute, we now look round to find the next level of integration. What variety of spaces is there that could yield a system higher than space? Surely none! We seem to have come to the end of sensory integration in a system that embraces all the senses and leaves no room for complication.

This unwelcome conclusion would compel us to suppose that the whole range of cognition cannot spring from one source in sense. A new beginning would have to be made from which perception, conception and the products of conception would emerge. There would, therefore, be two sources in cognition—sense and knowledge, a conclusion familiar in the history of mental philosophy, but as unwelcome and impossible now as it ever was. Desire for the unity and continuity in theory that the whole range of cognition seems to reveal in actual use, would force us to reconsider our course to see where we had gone astray from the true line of complication. If our beginning and first steps are as sure and firm as they seem on the whole to be, we should not have to search far for it.

In fact we have already caught a glimpse of it in the words "What variety of spaces is there?" of our first paragraph in this chapter. We found it useful to consider the integration of space first of all in its general character, just as we studied all the integrations as general types of process appearing in all the senses. But we have had present with us all the time the obvious truth that distances, intervals, and motions do not fill up the whole extent of our fields of sense at any moment. They appear only in so far as they happen to be elicited by stimulation. And usually there is only a limited array of them at any time. Pain, hunger, thirst, temperature, taste, smell and hearing are usually aroused only in fragments and at intervals of time. The field of vision is always full of sensation—an exceptional feature, as we have already noted. But distances, forms and motions within that field have all the same fragmentary and occasional character as in the other senses. And the distribution of clearness over the field makes the periphery more or less inactive without them. In stereoscopic vision our attention was specially drawn to the fact that only a limited block of solid figures is formed at any fixation, beyond which its unity merges into double images. These may draw the attention, when fixation will change, so that the block of stereoscopy is transferred to another centre, as it were.

The generalising, extending, functions of conception and imagination, with which our human experience is so richly garnished, incline us to suppose that in thus seeing into the solidity of vision at some one point, we are really looking there into a vast unity that is actually present to us as a whole, unlimited, indefinite, infinite. And the speed with which we change our fixations, that are undisturbed by the rapid blurring of retinal impressions between them, supports us in this belief. Without some careful study of vision, it is usually difficult for us to see how limited the vision of any moment is. We have to persuade ourselves to strip from it all this apparent infinity lent to it by thought and memory, so that we may the better capture an impression of its momentary fragmentariness.

But vision enters so intimately into the composition of our human space that, having so restrained our imagination in dealing with the tridimensional forms of vision, it is easy to repeat the discipline for the spatial contacts of vision and other senses. Thereby we soon realise that our sensory experience at no time deals with a single vast space or with total space in general, but only with a particular fragmentary space ; and that, in our sensory experience as a whole succession, there is not merely one space, but there is a vast, an infinite, number of spaces. From our advanced, philosophical or logical, point of view, we call these spaces fragments of space, since each one finally takes its place in, or relation in our minds to, the single whole of space of which we usually think. But as a matter of fact these (small) spaces stand in our sensory experience as entirely different, distinct, spaces. They may later come into conjunction with one another; and the processes of sense are apparently arranged for us so that the spaces we form will be apt to conjoin with one another. But to begin with, they are as separate and distinct as our concepts are. No one supposes that our concepts are from the beginning all delimited regions of a vast conceptual fluid that forms, as it were, a single ocean of generality. And yet concepts are gradually being arranged into a vast scheme, as science progresses. Mathematics shows us brilliant examples of this arrangement to form continuous series or wholes. Why then should we almost inevitably assume that the spaces we experience are from the start but tiny rooms cut off from space "überhaupt"? Surely only because sensory space lies lower down in our experience amongst the integrative processes that are more completely at our human command. We tend to ignore the work we have once upon a time done to link them into systems so well knit, that they seem to be continuous and to contain no component fragments.

Let us glance around our sensory experience at any moment, seeking out the spaces it brings in so rapid succession. I notice the articular feeling of my hand with the pen it holds, how it moves from left to right, oscillating rapidly as I write. I follow its spatial form to my shoulder, being aware from instant to instant of the space included by the curve of my left arm. My attention passes to the chair I am sitting on which gives me a sense of the angle of my trunk and legs, reversed successively at my knees and ankles. I see a chair: it is a seat, arms, and sloping back; I have to imagine the rest of it to realise its whole spatial form clearly: it invites me to turn round and to fall down on to it, putting my elbows down on its arms. I see a row of drawers on the desk before me. They suggest their motion forwards, to which my arm would move out in anticipation. Above them are spaces which invite me to pull papers out and push them in again. And so on. Every object I see as a spatial thing has its own form conveyed to me by vision, articulation, or touch ; and it is bound into a peculiar whole along with movements of my hands and limbs, which with it are ready to compose spatial motions and figures. It is not one desk that is before me, unless I turn my thoughts to its whole shape and matter, which I occasionally put my shoulder to and shove from place to place on the floor. It is rather an infinite variety of bits of spatial things that in some marvellous manner all fit into one another physically. They need not, of course, therefore fit into one another equally in my experience or thoughts. Each one of these chunks of space, in fact, rather runs out into indefinite sensations that my actual or incipient movements no longer reach or follow at the moment, even if they could follow them if I wished them to do so. Possibly the build of my desk would prevent this.

We have, therefore, a wealth of experiences with which we can pursue the complications of integrations. These little spaces are the product that the space integration provides for us : and we shall expect to find that two or more of them will group themselves uniquely together to produce the next level of integration after that of space. Our present task is to see more clearly what it is that these spaces actually are functionally in our experience. And our suggestion now is that they are identical with the simplest and most primitive form of perception.

And this is very nearly what has been commonly thought to be the meaning of perception. We may discount the use of the word that sees in perception nothing but a complex sensory mass of any kind which we use, and learn to recognise, without any further, or final, analysis of it, e.g. timbre or the " localisation " (binaural position) of sounds, or the like, especially in so far as the mass is held to contain nothing over and above the elementary products of its analysis. If such mere grouping is characteristic of perception, it would be more scientific to use some such term as sense-group instead of perception. But mere grouping cannot be an important functional characteristic. For we often group together a number of sensations, for example, all the spots of warm or cold excited by an areal stimulus of temperature on the hand (or the areal sensation that all these "sensations" constitute by aggregation). If there is a special difference between that and a tone-clang (or an instrumental tone, as we have called it), the difference must be more than a difference of the effect upon our action or attention; it must be a difference in the sensory complex itself, an integrative unity and product. If not, there is no difference on the sensory side and there is no difference between sensation and perception as experiences. We have not made any distinction between a pure tone and a clang (or timbre) as sensations; the one is relatively single and simple, the other is rather a complex or aggregate. But both as volumic figures have much greater similarity than this distinction would suggest, as we have seen. We have given these differences names that seemed generally suitable to them: and perception is not one of them.

Perception generally implies something more than "objective" sensations and their groupings: it seems to reach out beyond them to the thing, to an "it" unnamed and unthought, but still "perceived," that we have separated to some extent from its sensory surroundings and made our own by action. Perception is "taking through, or by means of." Ception, or "taking," is the same as sensation, which is reception. In perception we have also sensation; but this seems to us to be rather a medium by which we reach a structure of which it is a part, but which nevertheless extends beyond it or includes this medium and other parts in a unity. And this whole unity is the "it" we experience in a percept. It is that which forms the primary nucleus of an individual object, that is so generically the product of perception. This reference to an object naturally tempts us to suppose that in perception we do somehow transcend experience or enable experience to move out beyond itself, as it were, to include a real object of the outer world, and to point to it. But it would be philosophically naïve to suppose that we ever do really get outside our minds to inspect real things in themselves. There are undoubtedly in the world a vast number of things that we cannot directly observe: we can observe only their effects upon us and our experience ; or, observing the occurrence of various events in our experience, we are led to refer these events as effects to causes whose nature we try to determine from study of the effects. All the objects of our observation, whether simple or complex, therefore, in which we observe events and changes that in conceptual cognition we can think of as effects, must stand within our experience. The type of such objects we are now concerned with is perception.

Now not only does perception involve this "it," but there is also a clear reference from "it" to the sensations it includes and from them to it. In so far as any one participant sensation so refers to, or is attached to, the whole or to another, it is pointing beyond itself. It is, therefore, the function of integration itself which endows our complex experience with an apparent self-transcendence. And clearly we must expect the complexity or "distance" of this reference or attachment as it were, to increase as integration ascends to higher levels. The far-reaching reference that points from ideas to real things of the world only takes full shape in the higher refinements and complexities of conception. But we see the first steps of its extension in the integration of perception beyond the immediate references to one another of (a) the two sensing spots that have a distance between them and (b) this distance or vice versa (which was our first or most primitive type of integration).

And perception, as for so many psychologists of recent decades, also involves the co-operation of action. The "it" is as much made by, or consists of, our action, as it consists of the objective sensations which also participate in it. And our inclusion of the "kinæsthetic" senses in the fields that contribute to the formation of a space would confirm this "motor" type of perception. Only we cannot mean by "motor" mere physiological motion. That may ensue from any kind of experience, and will make no difference to it whatever. The term "motor" must apply to sensations which join with others from other senses to form the space-fragment that is the perception. Nor can it mean merely "associated" experiences of movement or the reproduction of "ideas of movement," the type of empirical or genetic theory of position, localisation, and space that is frequent amongst psychologists. This type of theory points to the " motor " factor, but fails to account for the nature of the " association " in question or of the resulting space in systematic terms.

And, finally, of course, this space is not a mere space like that of a geometrical construction, devoid of any quality or intensity of sense and of all temporal data whatever. The sensations from the participant senses carry their qualities and intensities along with them into the integration. And these may be important guides to the spatial action that may ensue. But these qualities and intensities do not float out of their respective fields, as it were, to fuse with one another into some new or old, but different, quality. They remain as distinct and particular within the integration as they were before it. So do all the attributes of the participant sensations. There is no loss of being in integration, as we have already noted in previous chapters. The only change is the " emergence " of a new inclusive system of position-extents (or space) in which each of the participant sensations now stands or partakes, whereby its original positions, extents, figures, motions, etc., obtain a new meaning, as has often been said.

And differences in temporal attributes are carried along in the same way. When I see a chair that I may sit into, the action of sitting is a temporal figure as well as a systemic one. And the space of the (chair's) " it " may change progressively in my experience as I proceed to sit down into the chair. Various space figures become evident in my experience, as I sit down, from stage to stage of my action. Or a dog, pawing open a swinging gate, may have to get through in a certain time or be nipped. And yet the systemic aspects of this structure are the essential basis of the space figure, not the temporal ones. Here we merely see another instance of the fact, already noted, that any systemic integration may be founded upon successive, as well as upon simultaneous, sensations. Neither the simultaneous, nor the successive, aspect is the more important, of course. Both rather are identical, in spite of the presence of time extension in the one and its absence in the other.

Time, as we saw during our special study of it, does not

integrate beyond the simple intervals and rhythms of its dimension. It displays no variety of fields, unless each sense is a separate field of time, in so far it is not yet correlated with the other fields. But this correlation seems to be primarily systemic, not temporal. We form no higher structures of time with the differences of the intervals that may appear in different fields because of their different (physical) time-distances from the stimulating processes, as it were. The only value of the co-ordination of the times of different senses is the coincidence or difference of the time of their various sensations.[1] The dog must get through the gate in a certain time, or be nipped. The spatial figures involved in his actions do not differ greatly with different speeds of movement.

Temporal figures, therefore, enter simply into systemic integrations of any kind, so that we have spatial motions, as well as stereoscopic motions. Spatial motions may be internal to their space or they may involve the spatial figure as a whole. A percept may thus be said to be a piece of space-time, to use Professor Alexander's terminology (of course without the implication developed by him that quality and intensity consist of, or are, integrations of space-time. In the qualities and intensities of sensations there is no sign of any systemic or temporal basis at all).

The importance of the systemic basis becomes more evident as cognition progresses to greater complexity. For space then becomes more and more the non-temporal space of our thoughts. Or it has become so, at least : perhaps we are now reverting in the theory of physical relativity to a construction based upon percepts in which we retain the time figures, carrying them steadily onwards throughout our conceptual elaborations of space.

As the average mammal, excluding the primates, is in all probability incapable of any sort of conception, we should expect to find that perception, thus conceived, is the highest reach of their minds. We should, therefore, expect it to

[1] It is for this reason that Kant and others have said that time is the " form " of inner sense, space being the form of outer sense. Strictly, however, this distinction is tautological : it merely says that space is space and time is time, with their respective characteristics. What these are our text indicates.

consist of the experiences that we may attribute to the mammal in its most intelligent type of behaviour. We must, of course, expect to find a similar type of behaviour widespread in our own actions, though at a far lower level than our best. This kind of behaviour in the mammal is its "learning by experience" or "by trial and error": in short the "tricks" that it learns towards various individual constituents of its environment. These are all essentially spatial, even if only by the fact that the behaviour is adjusted to the object in its place.

We have already seen that much more of the animal's behaviour is the work of pure reflex action, than of ours. His walking, running, swimming, flying, etc., are not generally permeated by conscious control, as ours are, but only rarely and momentarily. The new-born chick gets up and walks, avoiding obstacles in its path, as if it were already trained to do so, just as our eyes blink to a rapidly extending shadow on the retina, as if we knew we had to avoid it. So we must think of the animal generally as running about in its world mechanically, only seldom coming to an "object" that is experienced by it as an object, as a spatial "it," which it must negotiate in some way: just as we, on a higher level of experience may take a leisurely walk, only seldom seeing anything that strikes our conceptual powers and still less our reason and inference.

From our previous study of space we have learnt that it is not formed automatically by some mechanism. It involves a great deal of work, of learning by trial and error, based upon the creature's own spontaneity of effort and movement. For it consists in the attachment of the parts and contents of "near" fields of sense (articular, tactual, muscular) to those of the "far" senses (vision, hearing, smell, etc.). The resulting trick is the frame or skeleton of the piece of space that is formed and that constitutes the perception. Not that the animal abstracts its trick movement from the whole or from the objective sensory data into which they link. The whole complex is a somewhat indefinite unit that can know nothing of the abstraction of qualities traditionally associated with the idea of perception, as exemplified by the orange, with its touch, taste, smell, shape, surface, etc. That scheme can represent only the highest and most finished grade of perception, if indeed it does not essentially involve the work of generalisation and conceptual abstraction. It represents, in fact, the generalised individual, rather than the primitive percept, which as such involves no combining of different historical perceptions at all, but only the formation of a functionally general, or stable, integrative complex.

An example in which an animal learns to perform an action with apparent skill and yet seems to behave with great stupidity thereafter will serve to impress upon us the vagueness and fragmentariness of its percepts. In one of Thorndike s experiments the cat had to learn to get out of the box by pulling down with its claws a loop hanging outside the box, whereupon the door of the box fell open and the cat was free. But after it had learnt to do this skilfully as soon as it was put into the box, the cat still went to the usual place and clawed for the loop even when the loop had been removed. It can have had no "free" idea (whether sensation or image abstracted from all other sensations or images), and no thought, of the loop. It did not perceive *the loop* as such, we may say. "The reaction," as Thorndike said, "is not to a well discriminated object, but to a vague situation, and any element of the situation may arouse the action." The loop was merely a part of the situation or of the block of discomfort (hunger, vision, impulse-to-claw-outwards), and resulting impressions of contact, resistance, etc., that were more or less vaguely correlated in respect of their systemic positions and their forms and changes, and thus formed a primitive percept. The impulse was not solely attached, as we tend to suppose by inference from our own experience, to the precise form of the loop as the abstracting eye of the mind sees it ; it was attached to a large visual mass containing seen forms of various kinds (not abstracted from one another), and some of these could lapse without seriously altering the practical function of that visual complex in the animal, i.e. without failing to induce it to go to the corner and claw-for-loop. But of course, if the complex were changed more than a certain amount, the situation would no longer really be present and the animal would not respond. But what precisely the nature of the situation is, it must be extremely difficult to prove experimentally.

We can gain further light on this primitive state if we look for an example in our own conduct. Many people understand very little about the mechanism of the simplest machinery. They do not even trouble to look at the parts of it. They learn how to use it by rough trial, aided by some simple verbal instruction or by imitation, but if anything goes wrong, they are quite incapable of repairing the defect. If the nut on the under side of the lid of a metal teapot or under the seat of a bent-wood chair loosens, it is allowed to unscrew gradually (" this is getting loose," they say), it falls off and is thrown away (" the nob of this lid has come off "), and the article is then " broken " and useless. Such an object must be a very vaguely defined percept in such minds. Parts of it that are not essential for use disappear unnoticed, and efforts are made to use the thing when its essential parts have gone. To the expert or observing mind this seems as stupid as the cat pawing for the loop that is not there.

The study of animal behaviour has made it abundantly plain how important the animal's own action or spontaneity is to the progress of learning. Next to nothing, in fact, is learnt apart from spontaneous impulses to movement. Passive manipulation is nearly useless. A situation must be brought about that prompts the animal to move of itself: and the outcome of this movement must by the luck of chance sooner or later be the satisfaction of some appetite or emotion. Sight and sound, etc., by merely varying together do not form percepts. Nor will these and passively felt movements of the body form them. There must be some current of natural, reflex, or other spontaneous action, into which these sensations of sight and sound, etc., as well as of the ensuing movements may run out and, in so occurring together, have opportunity of establishing contact with one another as sensations, so that this psychophysical process in turn may become a conditioning stimulus to the primary current of action. That simply means, in other words, that there must be a current of " energy " flowing, if any complex of sensations is to form a " condition " of such flow at all and so to participate in the energy that is flowing. All the parts of any psychophysical mechanism are autonomous and contributory of energy, of course. But the largest part of energy comes from the primary nucleus of instinct or emotion, and it draws into itself the smaller amounts contributed by the participant associated senses.

Of course, we may direct an animal how to learn by inducing him to go to the right place or by supporting him here and there and the like. That merely means restricting his chances of useless movement, not doing the required movement for him. It still allows him to make all the effort. Eliminating waste effort in this way is not harmful in these lowly stages of cognition as it is in the higher reaches of it. A child must often be allowed to search for itself, because it can be exercised in methodical foresight. The child has the conceptual apparatus for discovering the way of success ; the animal (or the child or man who is working at this low perceptual level) has only the chance of success, so that it is obvious economy of energy to decrease his chances of failure. This we may do in all cases where explicit training in methods would be useless, uneconomical, or merely unnecessary. It would be useless with stupid folk, uneconomical in many departments of school and factory work, and it is unnecessary very often in the routine of daily life.

In certain cases, however, animals that have regularly been dropped into a box, to be rewarded with food soon afterwards, do sooner or later drop themselves into it or jump in of their own accord. White rats did so after two hundred days, rabbits in a few days, as also racoons. These cases do not necessarily conflict with the principle of spontaneity. For as the animals were often fed in the box, the sight of the box can of itself prompt to movement towards it, an action that is already fully within the animal's powers. And spontaneity to movement which may occur just before or during the process of lifting must appropriate to itself whatever impressions accrue thereafter, so that manipulation is then merely the setting of conditioning stimuli to these movements when they next recur apart from manipulation. The animal then learns a new trick by itself ; and it is only a coincidence that it is the same as the previous passive action—the same and yet so different, since the animal merely goes to the feeding place and does not stretch itself out as if it were suspended in a hand, or the like.

After this discussion it is unnecessary to show that the earliest forms of perception will not involve any imagery. For imagery implies a very high degree of abstraction as well as considerable perceptual, if not also, conceptual elaboration. An image is one of the products of the progressive complication and associative connexion of perceptions. It cannot be a presupposition of the simplest perception, but a much later consequence of its refinement. The most that we can ascribe to the simplest form of perception is a reference from one part of the basis of its space to the other, so that if part of the whole complex is given alone it will facilitate the presentation of the rest of it. Animals that have been trained to come for their food at a signal show every sign of attention and preparation. Fowls attend to the person who usually feeds them and still more energetically to the bucket their food is brought in. Their natural tendency is to get as near to either as possible. The dog surely does not, in any form of idea or knowledge, expect the flow of saliva that follows the sight of food, any more than we usually expect it when we see green gooseberries in spring. But neither to the little mind nor to the big one are the flow of saliva and the other feelings from the mouth altogether surprising. In the dog they will probably feel " all right," as they seem natural to us, so much so that we never " think " of them at our meals. Your call to the dog then probably sets up some sort of expectancy or readiness for the food-situation (visual, etc.) as well as some form of appetite. The associated sign will constitute a greater motor disposition to the actions already associated with it, and so will tend to connect the seen food by changes of position (visual and articular in some sort of parallel) with the mouth and with the positional and formal values of the taste as well as of the smell sensations that are located about the nostrils and vaguely in the mouth. Whether these dispositions will actually lead to movements (or to glandular secretions) in their degrees (e.g. looking at the food, getting up and turning towards it, leaping, running, barking, etc.) will depend upon the amount of energy flowing at the moment by way of this perception. Hunger would give a big supply. If the salivary glands secreted, the sensations therefrom would add themselves to those of sight and so increase the energy directed upon the perceptual centre. So would each new impression associated with propinquity to the food (as when the animal sets out in search of it) or with the sight or smell or taste of it, and so on.

So there is every reason why we should claim that at some stage of mental growth—not necessarily perhaps in a certain low grade mind, but certainly somewhere between that and our high grade mind, and probably in degrees of directness and force varying with such development—the taste-touch of the food, its smell, and the other regular sensory accompaniments of its presence, along with the sense of hunger or perhaps appetite, become centred on one another, so that henceforth each one carries a certain significance adjunct to them all. We might then admit that though these sensations are thus centred, they are not associated directly with one another so as to arouse each other (as mental images, for example). Each will tend to revive the percept-space constituted by them all, of which the kinæsthetic products of the creature's own movements form so important a part. In many animals this reconstruction may be restricted to the actual recurrence of the contributing sensations. In those of a higher type, however, there may be some degree of redintegrative revival in advance of actual recurrence. For this is a process that must begin at some level of integration, and seems very definite in our conceptual level of mind. But none of the sensations contributing to a percept would independently revive any associated sensation. Each would pass, as it were, by the perceptual " it " to the associated motor impulses.

Apart from the spatial implications, which are too complicated for illustration, the process may be symbolised thus (Fig. 20). The call (to food) along with a ready appetite tends to greater activity along acquired lines of habit or effort (M). Hunger without the call makes a wakeful ear for the call, since the call's " it " has been aroused by the perceptual centre to which hunger has been by habit attached; the call will find its "it" already awake when it comes. Hunger will likewise make an open (o) eye for any visible signs of food, if, indeed, it does not of itself bestir to motion along the lines of habit. In the presence of weak appetite these signs will naturally have slower and shorter effects, because so much of the energy available for action has been withdrawn by the weakening of hunger or appetite. When satiety supervenes the tendency to feed may be replaced, by the impulse to bury the rest or by sufficient attention to "it" for the animal to defend it, if need be.

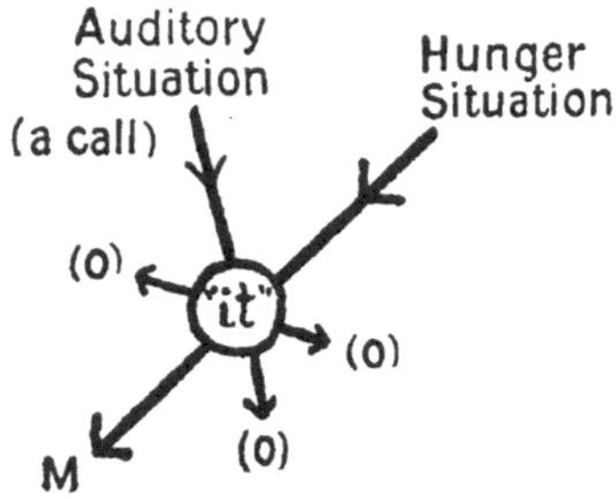

FIG. 20.

Thus far we have dealt only with perception as a typical process or with the single percept. But groups of percepts are often formed. We find it very easy to pass from one to another or to run through schemes or series of them from a single starting-point. A book or desk or a bicycle is a mass of parts, each of which we can handle appropriately and know. A door with an old and a new lock is to all intents and purposes a space of two parts for those who use it. One hand rises to the new lock, the other falls to the old one, each is turned in its own way, and the door-mass-of-space then moves "open." For many callers the door will be a space of one part, centred on the lock they by habit act towards (as *the* lock). Even a half-grown chimpanzee was found by Woodworth[1] unable to form a door-percept of two button-locks, although a door of one lock was completely learnt in three trials. The important parts were rapidly seized, for the chimpanzee soon limited her efforts to the two buttons. But presumably they existed for her only as one percept, while it was a matter of chance (1) which button of the two entered into that percept at any moment and (2) that the door was once opened by both buttons having been momentarily

[1] Ladd and Woodworth, *Elements of Physiological Psychology*. New York, 1911, p. 259.

left by her in the right positions. But monkeys have been found able to work a combination lock in which four fastenings had to be undone in a certain order.[1]

These examples serve to show us not only that percepts form complexes, but that animals readily learn to form single percepts, rarely or with great difficulty learn to form close complexes of percepts, while we have apparently unlimited power of doing so. The animal seems to need a special sensory sign for every trick. Every response it makes is a response to the situation in which it finds itself. It hardly learns to respond to situation *b* in a certain way (e.g. " turn the button and pull the door open ") because it has just responded to a situation *a* in a certain other way (" turn button *a* and then proceed to button *b* "). Its perceptual span of mind is only one percept big. Herewith we see how great a gulf separates us at this lowly stage from the animal mind. But the gulf is bridged more by the power of forming complexes than by that of perception strictly. The former is primarily a matter of memory, which, evidently beginning at the stage of perception, forms thereafter an ever more important part in the process of mind-building. It is one of the tasks of the science of animal behaviour to arrange the mammals in a serious of extending intelligence. Of those that can learn to work several tricks in a series, the monkey, the racoon, and the porcupine are notable examples. The porcupine can learn to operate puzzle boxes with four locks in a series.[2] The study of the development of perceptual ability in the child is a similar problem, which is partly covered and extended into the development of the higher processes of cognition in the familiar tests of intelligence of recent origin.

[1] Kinnaman, *Amer. J. Psych.*, 1902, **13**, 92 ff. 173 ff.
[2] L. W. Sackett, *Behav. Monog.*, 1913, **2**, No. 2.

14

CHAPTER XXI

RECOGNITION

EVERYONE knows that recognition is a special and peculiar kind of experience. You pass a face in the street and at the first glance you have a feeling which makes you say: "Surely I know that face! Who is it?" And then you spend time in searching the by-ways of your recent life to discover the place, situation, and time in which that face looked at you and engaged your attention in some dealing. When you have at last fixed it down, your mind is relieved and the process is complete.

A complex process like this involves much more than the mere feeling of recognition. If we reserve the term recognition for this first flush of arrest, which is the distinctive experience of recognition, we see that it is only the beginning of a long and complex cognitive process, involving spontaneous memory work, mental images, thoughts, feelings of doubt and certainty in their degrees, mental search, and so on. This is the broad difference between recognition as a specific experience and the very variable process of justifying it or of placing the recognised experience in its proper setting in space and time.

The process of justifying recognition clearly involves cognitive operations that are much "higher" than the specific process of recognition itself. The latter is an act that we should hardly hesitate to ascribe even to an animal such as the dog. You come upon him in one of his rambles in a general state of disengaged attention, taking his impressions for what they are worth as they come, and, at the half glance he bestows upon you as one of them, his eye is arrested for a moment, and he breaks out into rapturous greeting. When a visitor comes to the door whom he has learned to know a little, he will behave otherwise than he would to a stranger; but we cannot suppose him capable of searching in his mind to place the guest or to remember what favours he had received from him.

Thus we may place recognition as an experience next to perception. But how shall we explain the experience? Well, part of the explanation consists in merely placing recognition in the system of all experiences that we call the mind; and the rest consists in stating precisely what relation recognition bears to its next lower neighbour, perception. Now impressions that are very familiar are not recognised at all, especially if they appear in familiar surroundings which we already have in view. We do not "recognise" the usual furniture in our home or our usual relatives there or the utensils that are put before us from time to time. Their whole perceptual organisation is so clearly present to mind that it may be said to be continually present. Nor do we recognise objects that we see very seldom; there is a lower limit to our capacity; such objects have to be perceived anew. Recognition is intermediate; so that we might express its function by saying that, while the perceptual form in question must still be in existence, it must not be so actual as to be immediately accessible to incoming sensations. There must be some slight obstruction, due either to the age of the perception or to the great difference between the presentations of the moment and the usual circumstances of the perception in question; as when you meet a home relative in the crowded street unexpectedly. In the latter case the object in question would not belong to the group of objects or to the "situations" predisposed or revived in us by the impressions of the moment. Under these circumstances we may think that some peculiar collision of "percept-forming-under-the-force-of-presentation" and "percept-found-formed" takes place. This is the substance of the process of recognition in ourselves.

To form a clear notion of recognition we must try to think of the process as it would take place in a mind unlike our own, incapable of conceiving and reflecting in general terms, and not stored with an innumerable variety of percepts, but containing only a very few comparatively.

Let us return to the example of the dog that finds you in the street. His exploratory instinct—to invent a collective name for the moment—has him under control, and he has settled down to the even tenor of its actions. His generalised response to the humans in the street is more or less indifference to all (except boys, especially errand boys and " tramps," who both possess a subtle power of alarming him). You then appear. There is for long as you approach no response; you do not evoke a percept, or at least none of more than momentary duration. Gradually, however, you come within his range of clearer vision (usually not very many yards), or his attention is released from some other percept and you come within the range of his visual survey. There is the usual brief glance, which is arrested for an instant, then he moves forward a little, and, as more and more of you as his usual percept comes into action in him (including your response to him as a percept of your own), he bounds forward with rapturous greeting.

Our sympathy with the animal's behaviour would therefore lead us to locate the process of recognition just at, or after, the moment of arrest of glance, extending in time to include little more than the first movement forward, and ending just before the decisive actions of greeting begin. The process of perception at this moment falls into the traces or structure left by the you-percept. This in turn opens a course for the latently accumulating forces that bind the dog to you, namely, food-, comfort-, play-, and companionship-appetites, for the satisfaction of which in very appealing ways he is so dependent upon you. Not having been exercised since he last saw you or some other house-patron, during which time he has been bored long enough to gather energy to go on a ramble by himself, these appetites are strong, and only need the merest touch to spring into action. If the day were very hot, he would be lying prone in the shade and would not even raise his head for you. But now they are released, and rushing through this percept to which they are so strongly attached, they give rise to great energy of expression.

The process of recognition, we may infer, is that in which

a percept forming or being actuated in connexion with one set of energetic sources (appetite, instinct, etc.) suddenly finds itself running in the lines of a previously formed percept that admits an inflow of energy from some other such source. The energy supplied by the present percept alone could not possibly explain the sudden outburst of energetic expression. A new source must have been tapped in the animal itself. The present visual data sufficed merely to open the sluice of it. It is surely the inflow of these action-making forces through the percept as now sufficiently formed by the driving sources in action thus far, that constitutes the experience of recognition. And so all observational records can do no more than set down this first flush of recognition as a feeling of ease or of familiarity, a feeling of being at home, of being suddenly set upon smooth ways in a gradient, and so forth. But, of course, mere smoothness would not carry us far, nor would the force hitherto actuating us. If no other living spring were tapped by the impression that is the centre of recognition, it would be left merely as a thing of indifference, as far as our previous interests were concerned, or it would not be for them a percept at all. And the "hungrier" the springs now tapped are for outflow, the more vivid or intense will the experience of recognition be. If it is true that we do not remember unless we have a wish to, i.e. unless some source of mental energy is ready to revivify the memory, this is equally true of recognition, which everyone admits is a primitive form of memory.

A certain range of difference is caused by the degree of vigour of the percept as it has already been established. If it is recent and strong, recognition is not likely to be a distinct process, because then the structure of the percept is almost actual or conscious, and the purpose or appetite it usually serves has presumably been satisfied. Nor do we recognise things which immediately take their place as instruments of a continuous purpose or activity. When you take up your pen to write, you do not recognise the ink bottle before you put your pen into it, nor the blotting-paper when you come to the end of page. But if you turned the page of a book you were reading and found there a pressed and faded flower, you would probably recognise it ; for it would release the secret springs of the memory events that led to its insertion in the book. Or if you came upon a passage made familiar to you in lecture or recitation, you would recognise it still more evidently, for it would allow a current of thought and memory to intrude upon your present mental activity. And recognition is never so obtrusive as when the objects of a present activity tap springs of still active force in our minds, in other words when trains of activity cross in a common object.

When a series of smells is examined for the purpose of recognition, familiar ones give an immediate recognition that guarantees them to be right and requires no further mental activity than this. The observer need not pass beyond the moment of recognition even to recall the name or use of the smell. He knows at once that he could easily give these if required. It seems doubtful whether a mind lying or acting at the animal level would experience anything like this in passing familiar objects. Such a mind is neither thinking at the moment nor is it capable of the self-restraint or lack of practical purpose involved in the purely cognitive act of recognising and then of thinking "Yes, I know." The animal's recognising would result, not in a certainty of thought, for it probably has none, but in a sudden openness to associated impressions and an ease and vigour of transition to appropriate action. But this action implies the presence of a force driving to such action. The recognition merely means the tapping thereof. For a parallel example we should have to think of an animal playing say with a rubber ball that suddenly turns into a ball of bread that can be eaten, when there would be a sudden pull-up, sniffing, and then delighted consumption. If the appetite for bread were completely gone, it would not pull up at all probably. So we hardly recognise the postage stamps that delighted our youth : we hardly perceive them as passing things of the moment fully enough even to come near the individuality of the percepts of these early days.

When a percept taps a current of feeble strength, the "feeling" of recognition is less vivid and the mind has to move some distance before it comes to rest again. The animal proceeds to sniff at you—his best means of verifying a reference. When we think we recognise an odour, we try to get it into a memory-situation in which the actual sensation will play the part of a smell in our mental imagery. We sniff at the bottle as if we were in imagination sniffing at a bag of sweets, or cinnamon, or lavender, or as if we were sniffing around in a chemist's shop. And we continue till we find one such memory-situation that gives us a feeling of certainty and so arrests the mind. The term memory-situation here reminds us of the animal's failure to analyse its sensory situations. We verify our mental references by turning up the place in our "ideography," as it were. Sometimes, however, a recognition is so weak that it has not the strength to verify itself; it has the feeling of being ours, but no force flows into it to carry the memory to any conclusion.

These processes of ideational recognition in ourselves are based upon association. But it is often possible for true associations to be revived by present percepts (even when there is a definite purpose to recognise) without any recognition taking place. The force of revival seems to proceed entirely from the present impression and percept. There is then no tapping of a structure of mind out of which wells forward a force that carries us easily along and that constitutes recognition.

Conversely, there is a process known as false recognition, that occurs when one is "off-colour" or in a dreamy sort of state. Then, it may be, a scene that we have certainly never previously witnessed, some landscape or event in a region we never visited before, seems to be quite familiar or already experienced. False recognition is antecedently by no means improbable. For since in all psychophysical relations, everything depends upon the complex of mental processes set up and nothing upon the real events except in so far as they help to set up these processes, we can readily understand that the situation in question might be functionally identical with some previous one without really being the same, and without our necessarily being able to say in what parts or details the identity resides. For these events are commonly apprehended by us as "situations" merely, as far as recognition is concerned. And then a set of parts of a new situation might well be able to release the suspended interest that has survived from a previous situation in which it was rooted. And that we meet these illusions in our vague and less critical moods points all in this direction.

In this type of false recognition we have supposed that the main cause of the error lies in a genuine functional similarity of a new percept with some old one. But there are cases of false recognition that belong to the sphere of psychoanalysis, occurring very frequently in the patient and having no such genuine basis. They are chiefly due to a " desire " to feel familiar or at home ; and that desire is the expression of a starved or repressed (normal) appetite for at-homeness in other fields of experience. This banks up there till it bursts its bounds into quite inappropriate regions. Fundamentally, however, the scheme of things here is the same as before. Now, only, the merest trace of familiar conditions in the object is able to release a flood of bottled-up energy, so making a compelling sense of familiarity, of having been there before.

It has often been said that in recognition we compare the present percept with a former one. This usually means that we call up an image of the previous presentation. But experiments show that no such process is necessary, and in sure recognition rarely occurs. It would, in fact, be useless. For in sure cases we have already recognised before any such recall. And this we must really have done in any sort of recognising. For why should we try to verify by recall unless we have already had the feeling of recognition ? Verifying is only the transference to a surer recognition from a weaker one ; it is not the passage from recognition to something else. We can compare in memory without recognising ; and if we recognise and then recall and compare for the purpose of verifying, we only finally recognise, if we can recognise the recalled image instead of the presented one as being with certainty such and such.

Although recognition probably does not occur until the mental level of the perceptual process has been attained and has reached some degree of complexity, it seems fairly clear that other and " higher " processes such as concepts, judgments, memories, images, etc., can be recognised. This would probably lead us to the generalisation of recognition as a mental process, say as " x-process formed under one source of mental energy " tapping " x-process previously formed under some other source of mental energy still potent enough to fill it." Therefore, recognition would not so much be a specific link in the hierarchy of integration or of mind-building as rather a phenomenon generally characterising the specially cognitive integrations, a sign of the currents of action that cross mental structure in various directions.

In the human mind the feeling of familiarity is perhaps less pronounced than is the consciousness of the unfamiliar. A new experience arrests the easy flow of ideas and movements, for more work than usual has to be done in the perceptual process. By these signs we are aware of the unfamiliar immediately. But apart from the shocklike character of the process, which in sudden impressions carries us rapidly into the region of the emotions, there is no special type of experience or integration in unfamiliarity. This awareness in our minds is probably conceptual throughout ; in other words it is a sort of inference from the change in our current of ideas, etc. Besides at the pre-conceptual level we do not need an experience for the unfamiliar : the mere presence of a new impression is enough, for that has all its own peculiar potencies.

CHAPTER XXII

CONCEPTION

CONCEPTION may well be said to be the element of cognition proper. The term cognition has often been used as a general name for all the parts and processes of experience that reach from the elements of sense to the highest processes of thought. But it is also commonly used in a much more restricted sense, after which we can hardly say that a creature cognises, or is conscious, unless its mind has risen to the level of conception. Consciousness means verbally knowing-together, as does also cognition, while concept is the taking-together. Now, while we could hardly deny that the animal mind perceives in the sense of our foregoing exposition, the whole of the study of animal behaviour forces us to the conclusion that only the very highest of animals—those most nearly akin to ourselves—if any, do ever take percepts together so as to carry over and apply to one of them what it has learnt in connexion with another, and so to imply the occurrence in its mind of a process that might be called inference or reason or the appreciation of a feature common to a class of situations. On the contrary it can hardly even form a complex of more than one percept, but is limited to the response learnt in connexion with each situation. And this situation must be actually before it or no response is forthcoming.

The existence of a definite conceptual experience has been greatly debated, but there is very good evidence for its existence. It is denied by the ancient doctrine of sensationalism, which rightly looks upon sensations as the elementary stuff of all mind, but wrongly denies the occurrence of any form of union amongst them but aggregation. Thus nothing new beyond the elements of sense and residual traces (images) could ever emerge, even in the vastest mind. In the modern forms of this doctrine the apparent absence of sensations or their traces from many of the processes of thought that have been experimentally observed, is explained by the assumption that these traces become so fragmentary and fleeting that they usually pass (almost) undetected. Such a theory leaves us wondering how thought can still be so clear, although the stuff of it has become so attenuated, and why thought is so unlike sensation.

If all experiences were either sensations (even if we admitted feelings as the only exception), or aggregates of sensations, it seems clear that no experience could ever mean anything ; i.e. it could not refer beyond itself to what was not yet present but was implied, or was to be expected. It would just be itself and no more than that, self-contained as every elementary sensation is. Even if these experiences were associated in manifold ways with the same word, as the doctrine of nominalism supposes, that would not create anything functionally like a concept ; for we should then have merely the word in the form of some kind of sensation or mental image (trace of sensation) plus the experiences recalled by association with it. Those that were not revived by association would in no way alter our experience, for there is ex-hypothesi no kind of experience that means anything or is other than sensation.

By logicians a concept has been defined as a class of objects. Thus the concept of " chair " is the class of chairs, the concept of " three " the class of triples. This device saves the logician the bother of trying to find some property common to all the members of a class or to our perception of these members. The logician takes it for granted that we can recognise a chair or a couple or triple (of anything), when we meet one. He is not in the least interested in how we do so, but merely in the relations of classes to one another when they have been formed. There is no logical necessity for the class of chairs or of horses or of sixes, but, having been formed, they constitute stuff for the logician to work upon. Thus objects occur in the study of numbers that form a class called infinite numbers. Each one is formed in its own way, and they bear certain relations to other numbers, e.g. their part may be equal to their whole.

But there is no direct property or form, as it were, detectable in each, common to all of them.

It is not our business here to define logic or to show how it is connected with, and distinguished from, psychology. The latter is interested in the experiences " by which we think objects." And psychologically we must emphatically claim that if we can think of a class, we must do so in a special kind of experience. Truly, of course, this experience may not be something we detect in every member of the class or in the experience by which we perceive or think each one. Nevertheless, we must have an experience for the class, or else we should be able only to have its members in the mind as an aggregate (as the sensations of any indolent moment largely are) or as a matter-of-fact-sequence that we are not aware of as a sequence.

Experimental observation has shown that when classes of objects are formed, a corresponding experience appears ; or rather the emergence of this experience is the formation of a class. In rapid thought this experience stands for, or rather is, the class. And yet it represents neither any obvious property of all the members, nor of one member ; nor has this experience anything about it that looks like a sensation. But if need be, a representation or image of any member of the class may be forthcoming ; or there may be a sort of general image, a vague skeleton of the typical form of the members of the class.

The proper description of an experience of this nature is surely difficult, hardly to be solved merely by reading something off the face of it, as it were. But our previous studies of integration have provided us with a method of approaching it. That is, we describe it by tracing the resemblance it bears to other experiences and its dependence upon them, expecting that the experiences upon which it is dependent and of which it is the integration will also most closely resemble it. Now psychological reflexion has always looked upon the concept as a taking together or integration of percepts. But the percept is not itself an aggregate of sensations, but an integration of integrates of them. It binds them together and adds a new feature to their unity, thus being itself an experience which is linked continuously to, and so refers to, its basis. So too, doubtless, the concept emerges as a new experience upon the integration of percepts. And it will therefore not be itself any feature or property of any percept and yet it will functionally be, or stand for, any or all the percepts it integrates.

The development of the sensory cognitive system that we have traced out thus far, would now lead us to believe that the concept is but a further stage in the progressive integration of the systemic differences of sensations. If a percept is essentially a fragment of space, we can see beyond this one fragment a development leading to many others and finally to a whole spatial system embodying all our percepts, interwoven in their proper relations, such as science has so largely provided for us already. So we should expect the concept primitively to consist of a vaguely delimited fragment of a spatial structure, composed of the correlation and integration of a number of percepts. And the union of these we should expect to arise on the basis of their greater or less resemblance to one another. There can be no doubt whatever, that the primitive concept is a vaguely determined structure, not at all like the finished thing that enters into modern science and mathematics. It is just as it were the first glimmer of a common shape within many flickering forms. And it is generally agreed that the resemblance of situations to one another alone can bring them together, provided they first come into contact with some common interest or need in the creature. We have already seen how important this common interest is in the preceding stages of integration. We shall see its influence more clearly if we try to reconstruct the origin and function of an early concept.

It might readily be supposed that the sole function of conception is to enable us to think; and as thinking implies the occurrence and interconnexion of more than one concept, a single concept would be of no use whatever. Thinking is certainly one of the most important products of conception. But it is obvious that before we have many concepts, we must have one. And we may safely state the à priori rule that nothing comes into existence without thereafter changing in some manner under the influence of the forces that act upon it, so that everything has a function. What then is the function of a single concept?

What "good" would its first concept be to a child? We may suppose that many percepts have been formed in connexion with the appetite for drink: feeding-bottles, cups, spoons, tumblers have all been bound to the need for drink and to the movements required for the use of them in some way or other, since the child began to awaken mentally. They have also been bound to the sound of the word "drink" spoken by the nurse. Finally they are "concepted." Each gets a new meaning. From doing the "stupid" trick of getting its mouth ready, while the sound "drink" associatively stimulates its salivary reflex, the child becomes inspired, as it were. The particular features of each drinking trick are now accessible from one another: the child that has learnt only to help to grasp a cup, will "want" to grasp a spoon or fork. And the force of the associative sound "drink" must be grealty multiplied, since all occasion for the inhibitory interaction of its association to different percepts is now gone. And appetitive energy flows into the present action from all the other latent percepts that have become bound together in the new concept. So we may expect the child soon to make some show of saying this word, or, if it has previously learnt it trickwise, now to say it with greatly increased vigour and interest. Once the word has been thus connected, it will be brought forth on every subsequent occasion of drinking that has been similarly connected with the concept. And every item of action or meaning that reaches the concept through any one percept will rapidly appear with any and every other that follows—in spite of their differences.

The positional nature of the concept is not so distinct as to be beyond doubt. But it is by no means unapparent, and recent theories of thought that affiliate themselves to the results of the physiological analysis of action point towards a notion of a positional kind (the psychical correlate of the "final common path"). Concepts often seem to be stored "in our mind" like specimens in a vast case of pigeon-holes. They seem together to make up a system in which we can look around and search. In fact, order and arrangement seem to many to be the gifts of conception alone. It has often been thought that the elements of sensation of themselves have no positions, and form no relations (or integrations), but that only the activity of the organising intellect gives them these. This, as we have learnt from our close study of sensation, is a mistake ; but the view shows that, if concepts are not the source of all order, they at least seem to have order amongst themselves. But it by no means follows that the description of this ordinal character, and still less of the system they form together, is an easy task.

And if it was difficult in the perception to know what sensory parts were essential to its individuality so that their absence would leave the animal unresponsive to the situation in spite of the presence of the motive appetite, it must be far more difficult to know what features of the various percepts form the connecting similarity between them. We have an almost proverbial example in the child's " papa." This word as spoken by the child is first a " trick "-response, whose exciting situation is more or less uncertain ; then it surely becomes a trick-response to a situation in which the real papa probably figures as a matter of fact, but not, of course, cognised as that individual by the child. Thus the response will be called out by any object that resembles the real father, just as a dog that has learned to " beg " promptly will beg to anyone he meets who has food in his hands, provided he is not restrained by any circumstance. Later on in many a child the word " papa " may be used for a time merely to signify a man, after the child has learnt to distinguish men from one another, i.e. to adjust its trick-response differentially to different men. But what features of these men secure their inclusion in the class " papa " ?

Clearly amongst early concepts there can be nothing like " definition." This is only possible in a very late stage of conceptual development, when concepts have been formed in myriads, when complexes of them, judgments, and many other processes of thought have wrought them into finished form, so that we can say that the members of a certain class are such as contain in themselves as parts, qualities, properties, or functions, members of all the classes *b*, *c*, *d*, etc., in certain relations to one another. We have only to ask a child or a laymen in any branch of knowledge or practice to define any object familiar to him, e.g. cat, rabbit, bush, chair, flower, to know how vaguely delimited the distinguishing marks of it are. And yet these concepts may be used very skilfully.

We can now apply to the concept the results of our discussion of the association of sensations in perception. The linkage of percepts to concept will doubtless arise primarily upon the recurrence of similar but different perceptual processes in close proximity in time to one another and under the motive force of the same appetite. Thereby adaptation of the response to each percept becomes fluent while the differences of the percepts eliminate or greatly weaken from their " situations " those parts that are merely associative in them but not distinctive of them. As the forms from different senses are correlated in perception, thus emphasising without strictly delimiting one another, so the space-fragments of percepts, by being severally connected with the same responses, will functionally interpenetrate one another, as it were, emphasising or defining still more clearly the essential forms. Thus the concept becomes clearly a step on the way to increasing abstraction of forms. Its new phase of experience we may call the " a " experience, to indicate the meaning " one of," as against the restricted intent of the percept (" it ").

But in the concept the various percepts will not be accessible directly from one another. The male visitor does not call up in the child an image or other representation of the father, but evokes the responses and openness (to usual impressions) that the father prompts. And this is just how the concept usually functions in the course of ordinary thought. The a-ness applies to that skeleton of forms that, so far as it is delimited, is common to the various percepts ; it arouses the appropriate responses directly from and through these, and initiates the preparedness for various features not yet actually presented, but frequent in previous experience. In rapid conceptual work only the a-ness need be revived. But this limitation presupposes that conceptual processes have become so frequent that many relations have been established between them, that movements may be made amongst these relations without time being allowed for the responses to take place that are attached to the passing concepts. Such operations would not occur at all in the early stages of conceptual activity when only single concepts occur and that rarely.

Various attempts have in the past been made to show precisely in what manner percepts must interpenetrate one another so as to constitute the essential experience of conception. One of the most notable of them is Galton's notion of composite images. The now familiar composite photograph forms a material analogue to these. A dozen faces equally impressed upon a photographic plate or print make up a figure in which all common parts are clearly shown, while variant parts are visible according to their frequency in the twelve. The result is usually a very beautiful representation of a type.[1] But it is obviously still a single individual face, not a general face, or a face as one of a class. So however much of this kind of composition of images may occur in the mind, the essential feature of the concept—its generality, cannot consist merely in this. It was pointed out long ago by Berkeley that there can be no general image of many sets of things, e.g. of triangles. It is not necessary for the beginnings of conception that there should always be one ; for triangles are not amongst our earliest concepts and there may be many ways of making up a concept after we have been well provided with the earlier concepts and their relations.

But of simple material things there can be, and there frequently are, such general images. They are often found in introspective studies of thinking. A snake may be given by a wriggly line, a quadruped by a sort of oblong stool with legs at the corners, a vertebrate by a row of beads running into a blur of parts, and so on. Thus, the concept of a chair in its primitive form may well be a skeleton of the spatial form common to chairs, a raised level with a back or three-sided frame above, and props below. This would be but a restriction of the spatial form of the percept, already sketched for this example. And the general " chair " might well be this spatial form (embodying a similar skeleton of response in the form of articular sensation) in relation to the fuller spatial form of the percept of

[1] Cf. G. Treu, *Ztsch. Æsth.*, 1914, **9**, 433.

the moment. Thus the stuff of the concept would be a spatial form in relation to many percepts of ampler form, standing at different points of the system of percepts (i.e. of space, in the comprehensive meaning of that term), thus far formed by the creature in question. This spatial form would not necessarily correspond to any one full-bodied image (visual or articular); nor would it correspond exactly to any simple property of the chair as a material thing; but it might well be a vaguer and qualitatively less distinct (because primarily) spatial form. So it would be a property rather of the chair as apprehended and built up in our sensory experience. Possibly this sort of thing is implied in the many reports of vague forms of kinæsthesis recorded in experiments upon thought by Titchener and his pupils. Only it would not be merely a case of simple kinæsthesis, i.e. of a simple articular image, but it would be a case of a spatial image or better simply of space—which we here take as an integrate of vision (or other sense) and kinæsthesis (chiefly articular sense) together in a unity of which the new feature of space is the essence. If we have to define a triangle as the space bounded by three straight lines, the process becomes very much more complicated, but not radically different. Now the concept is a spatial form put together in successive parts and more cumbrously, but still in its fullest realisation a spatial form. In rapid thought we do not usually need to reach this fullest form of it. It is enough if we take it up at any point with the awareness that we are on familiar ground and could if need be carry it out fully.

It is thus easy to see how early concepts always contain in a prominent place within themselves the purpose of the objects they group. And so this purpose—its spatial usefulness—is readily made the differentia of the object by the child. A chair is for sitting on: a knife for cutting: a ball is what you throw, etc.

We have now reached a stage where it becomes impossible to move forwards without sketching vast fields of investigation in a few sentences. Between the simple and primitive process of perception that we find in the animal capable of learning a trick and the first signs of conception there lies the whole field of animal psychology. For its methods and results the student must be referred to the special treatises. The end and aim of this science in general must be to analyse all forms of animal behaviour, to grade them in their degrees of complexity, and to arrange the animals according to their degree of intelligence—the complexity of their percepts, the numbers of these they form, and their basis in sensation, etc. Thus we shall gradually learn how the bridge of mind that separates the vast bulk of the animal world from ourselves and our nearest kindred in it has been crossed. We shall learn the conditions that lie at the root of the higher grades of mind, and that we have carried on with us to form the structure of mind we share with animals, and that bears above it all that is our peculiar birthright. But we may feel sure that these higher levels rest and have grown upon foundations of the same type as those we find in the animal mind, but that differ from them only in their greater breadth and variety, not in some mysterious power that has been granted to us after a late stage of development as a divine gift as it were, and that has no organic basis in the lower reaches of our minds. If there is such a power, it is merely that of association, which, however, is not unknown in the animal, but that in ourselves is only far more rapid and fluent.

And behind the first steps of cognition lies the whole vast field of the psychology of thought, that has hardly yet been grasped even in the roughest scheme. Much experimental exploration and theoretical labour must be done ere we can hope to lay out satisfactorily the parts and processes of this great field, surely very much greater than we have ever yet supposed. Precise formulation of the nature of the concept can only be expected when we have reaped the results of this study and have carried many of its lessons back to the springs of our exposition as simple facts and postulates. This method has in the field of sensation led to the formulation of the attributes of sensations—notions which have so much helped to guide us through the mazes and variations of the different senses. But we can now see more clearly than before, how vague and ill-defined are the beginnings of conception, how much work has to be done ere we reach the precise concepts of the adult human, and especially of the scientific, mind, how the process of abstraction begins in the mere integrations of percept and concept themselves, and how sense through them runs smoothly and continuously into intellect. Everything that we can distinguish in sense is already there from the first, but it is only by the elaborate work of conceptually guided perception and abstraction that we can attain to the specific analysis of details, i.e. to the conceptual apprehension of them as parts of sensory data. We do not begin with a world of blurred and vague psychological realities that our thinking and similar higher powers of mind somehow reduces to clear-cut definition. It is only our conceptual processes that become more and more adequate, as they develop, to grasp and portray all the differences of sense that exist.

Of the conditions that enrich the sensory basis of the human mind and so provide the greater wealth of material by which it attains levels beyond those of the animal mind, probably the most important are the functions of the fovea, of accommodation and of static stereoscopy and the development of a delicate skin and prehensile hands. All these make in some way for a differentiation that is the first form of abstraction. The fovea refines and distinguishes positions and forms, while accommodation sharpens the objects of attention and dissipates the rest; stereoscopy adds a new character to a group of forms that may persist for indefinite periods of observation; delicate skin gives greater sensitivity to variations of pressure, and the prehensile hand implies a very great refinement in the positions and forms of the derived articular sense. In the hand this becomes a fine mobile tridimensional sense that, like the stereoscopic eye, can go round and through things, so almost isolating them from their surroundings. At the same time the articular sense is the conscious correlate of action and of the individual's share in his experiences. It represents the self at its lowliest stage perhaps; and, as we have seen, it makes possible the integrations of percept and probably of concept that are the beginnings of intellect—so private and inward a power that it has often been held to come towards sense from another region altogether. Thus we come into touch with the results of biology[1] as well as with the recent tendencies of thought that have been inspired by the later work of the physiology of reflex action. But these motor theories of consciousness, right as they are in stressing the rôle of action in making mind, commonly neglect to show how action enters into the data of sense to integrate with it and so build up psychical mind-stuff. Without this counterpart of movement in mind-stuff we cannot see how any physical or physiological process of movement can build up mind.

The size and complexity of the brain are correlated with the complexity of intelligence, so that it would seem that physiological factors must be responsible for the development attained by any mind. But we can bring these physiological factors in two ways into relation to the sensory basis of mind: (1) in respect of the variation of the elementary sensations that we here take to be the basis of the cognitive mind, and (2) in respect of the functions of retention and association that as such do not add any sort of element or complex to the mind, but only extend or retain what is already offered as sensation or has been integrated out of sensation. We are often inclined to suppose that many animals have finer senses than man. But for the upbuilding of mind, we must discount whatever advantage they have over us with regard to differences in the quality and in the intensity of sensations. For these two attributes, as we have seen, show practically no traces of integrative process. There will probably be little difference between us in the matter of the temporal attributes. That leaves over only the systemic attributes as the line of variation that is in all probability the most important for mind-building. And, therefore, we can understand how important the presence of a good articular sense as well as good vision must be for facile space-formation, i.e. for perception and its product conception. From this point of view the probability that the human mind is best endowed with the sensations requisite for mind-building seems far greater than in a general view that reckons all differentiation of sensations as equally important.

[1] Cf. G. Elliot Smith, *Essays on the Evolution of Man*. Oxford, 1924; especially Chapter III.

CHAPTER XXIII

CONCLUSION

SURVEYING the whole ground we have thus traversed, we can see that the mind has both a perpendicular and a horizontal structure, so to speak. The perpendicular structure is displayed in the system of integrative levels sketched in the Tables given above (pp. 65 and 151). We may now complete them by continuing the line of development that ended in stereoscopic vision into percept or space-fragment—(recognition)—conception—ideas, judgments, and thoughts. The horizontal level may perhaps first be traced in some of the sensory illusions, if there is interaction between the elements of form apart from all physiological distortion and from reactions of higher mind upon the senses. But at the best such interaction is still problematical, and until the integrations of perception and conception are reached, its effective force is small indeed. To make it evident the action of memory is needed, and then the horizontal level begins to vie with the perpendicular in importance and activity.

Thus the mind may be symbolised as a series of concentric spheres, the successive surfaces being: the elements of sense, their simpler integrations (form, motion, time), and the tridimensional complication of form, the correlation of the senses in the spatial fragments that constitute percepts, conception in its primitive form, and then all the refinements of thought still so vaguely analysed and discriminated. Over these surfaces, connexions occur between the threads of complication that travel inwards. The innermost sphere is that vast system of activities that we call cognition proper, whose elucidation is alone a task awaiting the energies of some efficient student of the experimentation of recent decades and the analyses of philosophers of all the ages.[1] It is this inner sphere that gives man's mind its scope and power. But we need not suppose that without it mind is not really mind but a blind mechanism; or that even with it we have learnt to transcend the limits of mind itself. The animal mind differs from ours not in a lack of sense or cohesion, but only in a lack of concepts and all their systems of interaction and grouping. We "see," only because we have that much more than the animal. But this conning tower rests on the ground on which things roam that also see, though less far at once, and more face to face, than from above, over many things together. And the cohesion of our concepts and thoughts is essentially as limited and continuous, constituting action over a distance as little as does the cohesion of our emotions or of the animal's perceptual cognition. In supposing that we penetrate so very far outwards from ourselves, we do surely mistake quantity of things seen for depth of vision.

Our mind is true in its actions, setting us into connexion with a real world, primarily because it is founded on so many elements in sense, each bringing its own contribution, which nevertheless shows itself capable of harmonious conjunction and co-operation with those brought by the others. The world the mind reveals is real because the mind itself is a real world full of vital activities, each linking vitally and intimately with the rest.

This is, in fact, a brief statement of the relation of mind to matter from the psychological point of view. As the result of our study of nature, life, and mind, we must look upon mind as a vast sphere of activities that is surrounded on all sides by the rest of the universe, acting and reacting upon its parts. Forces from the physical world stream into it and set it moving, and forces of the mind stream out making physical things move in turn. Of course, we must not suppose that before all experience the "empty" mind is a substance any more than empty space is a substance. The mind has to be built up from its elements

[1] I would refer the reader to Spearman's admirable work: *The Nature of Intelligence and the Principles of Cognition*. London, 1923.

before it can be said to exist, just as a living body has to amass its parts that proceed from the progressive division of its original germ. The problem of the origin of these elements we may ignore for the moment. And the problem of the persistence of the forms of integration of the mind that have been once constituted by the integration of its sensory elements—a persistence that is the primary fact of memory and thinking, opens up vistas that can hardly be surveyed from the present outlook of physical and physiological science. Their reduction to the simple physiological hypothesis of re-excitation of neural structures, however important and satisfactory as a partial solution (on the material side), does not yet allow of translation into terms sufficient for the psychological side. So then the forces of the physical world stream into mind (constituting its elements and their powers of integration) and out of it again, just in the same sense as they may be said to stream "up" into the world of life (constituting its elements and their powers of integration) and out of it again.

This does not in any sense imply that we ever get outside of our minds, as it were, so that we might see them and the physical world in a comprehensive glance. Such powers are reserved for the angels in Prof. Alexander's figure of speech. Our direct view is limited to the region of our own mind. We are conscious of its activities, or we simply are its activities, in all their various forms—knowing, feeling, and sensing. But these make up quite an extensive region in which with our high powers of cognition we can compare and connect one part with another. And so we find streaming into our sphere of mind actions of the most variegated patterns, that could not be set down as typical of mental process as such, and that therefore are not due to the structure or integrations of mind in itself. They are therefore variable forces, practically important as such, strangers as it were, gifts "from outside." It is our knowledge of these patterns of activity that justifies us in assuming (as the philosophers say) the existence of a world beyond our own minds. The unsophisticated mind surely does not assume at all. These changing intruders simply are for it intruding (outside) forces with which it must deal or perish. So the external world is simply that which is beyond the boundaries of the individual mind. It is the medium that embodies the forces of which these incoming activities are the result or continuation.

Thus we see that psychology need in no way incline to an account of mind that makes the world fantastic like the dreams of a maniac. Study of the elements of sensation does often give this sort of impression. Physical science has made us familiar with the idea that material things are colourless, soundless, tasteless, masses of particles in a state of violent agitation, and that all these qualities that make up the beauty and light of the world for us exist only in our own minds. The physiological study of sensation carries this distinction forward into the brain, so that psychology, whose task begins with the elements of sensation, seems to have nothing left for its consideration but a negligible phantasm that cannot be affected except through physical means, and is therefore of little use. Thus many recent philosophers have been strongly inclined to reject the whole idea of the universe that is based on this distinction. For every one of us the world is really a world of colour, sound, weight, smell, cold, and warmth. It is a world of space and time, solid and rhythmical, teeming with truths and most suggestive of errors, glowing with beauty and distracted with the conflict of good and evil. If we follow the results of science, must we take all these " values " as evanescent phantasms ? The conscious tendencies of these industrial centuries have led strongly in this direction. Values have largely been left to their chances of survival in the individual, when, of course, the selfish ones naturally predominate over those of a general or " higher " nature which the inherent nobility of each person protects. But there are many signs that the world of values and all its immediate psychological substructure is attracting the genius of scientific minds to its study and promotion.

Efforts have been made towards philosophical reconstruction that look upon colours, sounds, and qualities generally as a part, if not the sole stuff, of the physical world. The drawback of this outlook is that it is merely the converse of what it is intended to supplant. Only in it the physical world is now the phantasm. Molecules, atoms, and electrons are now merely theories, constructions that are nothing but a useful shorthand for describing large numbers of such phenomena as the qualities of sound and colour. Any such form of modern realism is surely not so satisfactory as is the realism of modern science. For while, in the latter, mind is the phantasm, in the former both sides take on a phantastic appearance. Not only do the notions of science become mere constructions, a shorthand for clouds of (mainly) visual phenomena, but the world of mind seems also to be nothing but an insubstantial drift of incoherent sensations, devoid of any basis of permanence. The inner world seems to lose its stability because its basis is drawn from under it. Like Berkeley, then, we must cry for a god to hold up all the colours, sounds, and tastes that the myriad lives of the world have had and have, and to bind them all together into a coherent world.

Modern theories thus seem to buy the primacy and reality of qualities, of truth, beauty, and goodness (if, indeed, these things are substantiated by them) at a dear price. Shall we not do better to accept all the results of natural science as real and valid as far as they now go? Our philosophies can only become real by penetrating the details of knowledge as positive scientific constructions. The study of mind impresses upon us the reality of all mental processes and values; and all our detailed knowledge of the mind's activities allows us to think of these activities as continuous with the processes and activities that form the physical world, surrounding mind and playing upon it. Our psychological study has impressed strongly upon us the fact that the distinctive unity of integration in mind adds to the substance of mind a phase that is the essence and distinction of each integrative level. So we can perhaps the more readily understand that we have no reason to suppose that the physical world is devoid of quality or of those binding forces that we see in our own minds under the guise of truth, beauty, and goodness. Physical science convinces us that the physical world has spontaneity of its own and is a coherent stable system with a great variety of forms and kinds of coherence.

These may be represented by the typical unities of proton, electron, atom, molecule, living cell, organism, etc. The coherence of these units must keep the physical world from falling into chaos, just as we all feel inwardly that the coherence we experience in truth or beauty or goodness and the various integrations of cognition and emotion form the stability and coherence of the mind's activities, so that the mind is not a mere whirl of sensations.

Thus we should conclude that we feel aware of these forms of coherence only within the sphere of mind, but while there is surely reality beyond this sphere, we are not directly "in touch" with it. We simply are not that part of the world and its coherences and processes. But as the rest of the world acts upon the mind, the processes in our mind can be brought into the pattern of the units and processes in the world outside. It is just the pattern of processes that can pass into the mind (ultimately in virtue of the presence of psychophysical parallelism), not the process itself, not its inner coherence. We can therefore know the external world only as a set of unknowns in certain relations, these relations being embodied in those systems of mind that are best capable of taking them over. Of these far the most important are space and time; for the qualities of our sensations show no signs of having any foreign (material) pattern embodied in them. And so the physical world seems to us to be a spatial-temporal structure of mere unknowns.

And we must go a step further still. For space and time as we feel them cannot be ascribed to the external world. Space and time, as in Kant's terminology, are evidently only "forms" of the mind. We cannot ascribe to the world the spaceness and timeness of space and time as we experience them, but only the patterns embodied in these matrixes. What the stuff of the external world is we consequently have no means whatever of discovering. Those who believe in a special vital process (vitalists) evidently believe that they can find out something more about the organisms we call living than the mere patterns of their distinguishable parts and processes. And they all spend much energy in expressing the fervent conviction that they can in this instance reach some sense of the inner coherence, purpose, or spontaneity of things. Life seems to be so very much alive. But the quest is as hopeless as is that of the perpetuum mobile. It is merely the attempt to get outside our own mind or our own being. We can never feel or know the spontaneity of the external world because we are ourselves just feeling and knowing, and we cannot be other than ourselves. Nor can we know the essence of its being in any of its parts. We can only take up into our knowledge the impress of its parts, a pattern that displays the connexions between them, and that is true solely in so far as we have striven to let no other object determine the impression made upon us than the one to which we refer.

And not only things, but minds must appear to us as patterns of parts and as the mechanisms which their changes constitute. For science rests upon thought, and thought lies in the cognitive level of mind, of which concepts are the proximate element. How can we expect to portray in this one level of mind the inner spontaneity and essence of all the other levels of integration? Only patterns can pass through different levels of integrations. We cannot even expect cognition to portray its own patterns completely in so far as they merge into the mere essence of thought. For thought cannot turn itself inside out as it were, in order to show its own nature the more clearly. Hence the futility of much of the discussion regarding the connexion between relations and terms. We cannot say whether a term in isolation seems to be the same as a term in relation to another, apart from merely standing in this relation. For obviously we cannot abstract the term from its relation and still leave it there. Nor can we describe in cognitive terms how a term is bound to its relation. The only pattern for the portrayal of this connexion that cognition has at its disposal is the very pattern in question. If we ever acquire a level of mind higher than cognition and integrated out of it, we shall then doubtless be able to give a better account of this connexion. But the method to be adopted then will surely be that which we have followed throughout this study, namely, to arrange experiences according to their resemblance to, and integrative dependence upon, one another, and to carry this out for the whole of mind, until we can see all its parts as members of a system of different levels and each typical connexion in any one level in its kinship of resemblance to the typical connexions found in other levels. Another level of integration would only extend this system, apart from the new essence it would bring to mind and the new capacities for portraying patterns that as a still higher level of integration it would contain.

Thus we see that there is an inner realism as well as an outer one. Any other part of mind is just as external from the point of view of conceptual portrayal as is the external world. A colour conceptualised is not again a colour; it is only the thing next to orange or the last of that series or the like. To get the colour you have to send your "gaze" back from cognition through perception to the colour itself.

As a characterisation of our psychological standpoint in general a summary of the preceding argument seems to point to some mechanistic type of theory. But this does not in the least imply that the processes of the mind are governed by material processes or conditions. They are bound together solely by their own mental laws and types of coherence. And the mind is imbued with its own innate spontaneity or drive. A mechanistic interpretation of mind implies, on the one hand, only the limitation of psychology to a portrayal of the elements and units of mind, their interrelations and patterns, and their series of changes, and, on the other hand, the exclusion of any conceptual understanding of the spontaneous, creative, decisive acts of mind. We cannot rationalise the inner life or being of mental events. All our science of mind points to some form of deterministic theory, in which any event of mind is determined throughout by previous mental events and conditions, leading finally back at all points to the world of external conditions. Only, all determinations other than these last are mental, not material. There remains at every stage of change the inner process which, though fully determined, is the burning focus of the event, and is the core of reality for the mind at the moment. A mental event would not be the same if we ceased to bother about it: it would be quite different if it were left to the care of its own conditions, so to speak, if it were treated as unimportant, so that the focus of interest of the mind passed to other parts or allowed entrance to other conditions than those in question. Every mental event as it proceeds at any moment always has its own warmth and grip, to which the self or the will seems to do homage. Thus though for scientific purposes one may be a good determinist, in actual life we all are voluntarists. We freely will in every event, even though we are then most bound by the circumstances of our choice. Our will is just this event thus governed by conditions, carefully held together by their most essential inherent relations. It is not an arbitrary act divorced from relation to all motive and purpose. Free-will is just the spontaneous and free or self-determined reality of mental process as against the unreasonable forcefulness of some partial set of conditions of a material appetitive nature.

Reverting, finally again to the efforts that philosophy is now making towards some form of realism, as against the subjectivism so typical of (modern) science, we can readily see that the whole sphere of cognition we have traversed can, if we feel so inclined, be reckoned to the "real" world, as distinct from that of the inner self, if there is such a thing. For conceptual cognition seems itself to be but a complication or integration of sensory space and that again of the systemic features of sense, which in turn no doubt have their parallel in the brain. And the physical disposition of the brain's activities depends upon the spatial arrangements of the stimuli that impinge upon the senses from the cosmos of events around us. Concept, thought, and reason are therefore but an outreach of the physical world, the variegated crest of the wave that our brain throws up in its ocean at the shore of our self. They are objective and real, as real as the eyeball or as the distance to the moon and its motions. But the difficulty in this sort of philosophy is that in our foregoing exposition we have postulated no self at all, and have had no need or use for one. There is therefore nothing subjective to set over against this world of reality of which the whole range of cognition is to be a part. There can surely be no need to draw a philosophical line between all reality and nothing: so we may leave the line where it has usefully been set and kept—between the "last" events of brain and the "first" events of sense, at least until we get some more cogent arguments for the existence of a subjective world (of self, or "ing" processes—sensing, thinking, etc.) than are as yet to the fore. The so-called argument against all idealism—that knowing and its object cannot be identical, is worthless: for no one is for a moment required to suppose that a concept (an "a" state) is identical with its reference to, and basis in, integrations of lower levels, who claims that there is besides the concept (or "a" state) no other state directed upon it (of concept*ing*). In other words, psychologically, thought may have an object and yet not need a separate process of thinking to own it or do it, any more than it needs a self to make it be a thinking. In any case the philosophical value of such realism seems small. For the only issue of it can be that after we have sated our hearts with this sort of realism, we shall begin to sorrow again for the great gulf that divides the self or the -ings from the last outposts of reality that face them. And besides, as we have seen, there is not, and cannot be, only one of these gulfs: there are many of them: every integration involves one. And who shall declare the kind of integration that a self so standing apart shall need? No, there can be no such one gulf. We learn from Kant's failure that there cannot be a complete cleft between intuition (space and time) and conception: we bridge the gulf, as far as may be, by seeing that conception is, and must be, itself essentially a complication of space. Nor can there be such a gulf between the matter of sense (sense-data or elementary sensations) and the "forms" of space and time. These must rest upon, integrate, and so share kinship with, attributes of the elementary sensations (systemic and temporal). And we must learn from these examples to carry our vision over the dark gulf that must somewhere appear for us (beyond sense-data), to things beyond, trying to learn from the system of mind how to think of them with greatest hope of truth. Then there will be no great break in the world at all. We can only strive to interpret the part of it that we are not, and do not really see with the inward eye, by the part of it that we are, and do so see, and by what we find streaming through this world of our own being from beyond.

INDEX